Delmar's Pharmacy Technician Certification Exam Review

by

Patricia K. Anthony, Ph.D.

Research Associate
The University of Arizona
formerly
Instructor of Pharmacy Technology
Tuscon Campus
Pima Medical Institute
Tuscon, Arizona

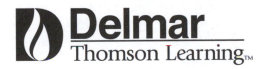

Albany • Bonn • Boston • Cincinnati • Detroit • London • Madrid
Melbourne • Mexico City • New York • Pacific Grove • Paris • San Francisco
Singapore • Tokyo • Toronto • Washington

NOTICE TO THE READER

Delmar Staff
Business Unit Director: William Brottmiller
Acquisitions Editor: Marlene McHugh Pratt
Development Editor: Marjorie A. Bruce
Editorial Assistant: Maria Perretta
Executive Marketing Manager: Dawn Gerrain
Channel Manager: Nicole Benson
Executive Production Manager: Karen Leet
Project Editor: Bill Trudell
Art/Design Coordinator: Rich Killar
Cover Design: Cummings Advertising/Art Inc.

JOIN US ON THE WEB: www.DelmarAlliedHealth.com

Your Information Resource!
• What's New from Delmar • Health Science News Headlines
• Web Links to Many Related Sites
• Instructor Forum/Teaching Tips • Give Us Your Feedback
• Online Companions™
• Complete Allied Health Catalog • Software/Media Demos
• And much more!

Library of Congress Cataloging-in-Publication Data
Anthony, Patricia K.
    Delmar's pharmacy technician certification exam review / by
Patricia K. Anthony
        p.   cm.
    Includes bibliographical references and index.
    ISBN 0-7668-0743-6
    1. Pharmacy technician's examinations, questions, etc.   2. Pharmacy
technician's outlines, syllabi, etc.   I. Title.   II. Title:
Certified pharmacy technician examination review.
    [DNLM: 1. Pharmacists' Aides Examination Questions.   2. Pharmacy
Examination Questions.   QV 18.2 A628d 1999]
RS122.95.A585   1999
615'.1'078—dc21
DNLM/DLC
for Library of Congress   99-25102
                                                                  CIP

Contents

Preface — vii

Acknowledgments — viii

Introduction — ix

Section I — Assisting the Pharmacist in Serving Patients — 1

Chapter 1 — Receiving the Medication Order — 3

The Medication Order — 5

The Medication Administration Record — 9

Comparison of Medication Orders in Retail and
Institutional Settings — 11

Chapter 2 — Processing the Medication Order — 15

Basic Terminology—The Dosage Form and Instructions — 16

Routes of Administration — 17

Interpreting the Order — 18

Dispensing the Correct Medication — 23

Comparison of Drug Dispensing in Retail and
Institutional Settings — 23

Chapter 3 — Preparation and Utilization of the Patient Profile — 27

Obtaining and Entering Patient Information — 28

Comparison of Patient Profiles in Institutional and
Retail Settings — 30

Chapter 4 — Handling Medications — 35

Use of the Manufacturer's Label to Correctly Dispense
Medication — 36

Packaging and Labeling the Medication — 37

Dispensing Liquid Medications — 38

Intravenous Admixtures and Injections — 41

Auxiliary Labels — 42

Chapter 5 — Proper Storage and Delivery of Drug Products — 45

Storage Conditions — 46

Preparation of Unit Doses — 48

Use of Pharmacy Inventory as Floor Stock — 49

Chapter 6   **Receiving Monetary Compensation for Goods and Services**   **53**

Methods of Payment for Pharmacy Services   *53*
Profit and Markup   *55*

Section II   ***Inventory Control***   **57**

Chapter 7   **Stocking the Pharmacy**   **59**

The Drug Formulary   *59*
Ordering and Receipt of Drug Products and Devices   *60*
Ordering Regular Drugs and Devices   *61*

Chapter 8   **Maintenance of Drug Products**   **65**

Maintenance of Drug Products in Inventory   *65*
Importance of Proper Storage of Drug Products
in Inventory   *66*
Handling Expired Medications and Drug Recalls   *66*
Drug "Recapture"   *67*

Chapter 9   **Commercial Calculations**   **71**

Cost and Markup   *71*

Section III   ***Pharmaceutical Calculations***   **75**

Chapter 10   **Fractions, Decimals, and Algebra Review**   **77**

Dividing a Whole: Using Fractions   *78*
Working with Decimals   *80*
Use of Algebra in Pharmaceutical Calculations   *82*
Rounding Numbers   *82*
Using Roman Numerals   *83*

Chapter 11   **Systems of Measurement**   **85**

Common Systems of Measurement   *85*
Ratios   *89*
Temperature Conversions   *90*

Chapter 12   **Using Percentages and Ratios**   **93**

Percentage as Parts Per 100   *93*
Using Alligation   *95*
Using Drug Concentrations Expressed as a Ratio   *96*

Chapter 13   **Measuring Equipment**   **101**

Liquid Measurement   *102*
Measuring Solids   *105*

Chapter 14   **Conversion of Solid Dosage Forms**   **109**

Converting Between Measurement Systems   *111*

Chapter 15 **Conversion of Liquid Dosage Forms** **115**

Converting Between Liquid and Solid Dosage Forms *115*

Chapter 16 **Pediatric Doses** **123**

Computation of Pediatric Doses—Differences from the Adult Dose *123*
Computation of Dose by Body Surface Area (BSA) *125*
Young's Rule and Clark's Rule *126*
Recommended Daily Doses (Safe Dose) *126*

Chapter 17 **Parenteral Dosages** **131**

Parenteral Dosage Forms *131*
Calculation of Parenteral Doses *132*

Chapter 18 **Intravenous Calculations** **137**

Administering Intravenous Medication—The IV Drip *137*

Chapter 19 **Intravenous Admixtures** **143**

Infusing Medications Over Time—The IV Drip and Admixture *143*

Chapter 20 **Calculation of Dose per Time** **149**

Calculating the Amount of Drug Infused per Time (Dose per Time) *149*

Chapter 21 **Bulk Compounding** **153**

Compounding Drugs by Procedure *153*

Chapter 22 **Math Test with Solutions** **159**

Section IV *Pharmacy Operations* *169*

Chapter 23 **Safety in the Workplace** **171**

Occupational Health and Safety Administration Regulations *171*
Disposal of Hazardous Waste *172*
Sanitation Management *173*
Spills *173*

Chapter 24 **Using Computers in the Pharmacy** **177**

Use of Computers in Pharmacy Practice *178*
The Components of a Computer *178*

Chapter 25 **Communications Within the Pharmacy** **183**

Role of the Technician in Communication *183*
Role of the Pharmacist in Communication *184*

Section V   Pharmacology   *187*

Chapter 26   Drug Nomenclature   **189**

Introduction   *189*
Proprietary Drug Nomenclature   *190*
Drugs That Affect the Central Nervous System   *191*
Drugs That Affect the Cardiovascular System   *197*
Drugs That Increase Pulmonary Ventilation   *203*
Drugs Used to Relieve Allergies (Antihistamines)   *204*
Drugs That Affect the Gastrointestinal System   *205*
Drugs for Use in Parasitic Infections   *206*
Drugs That Affect the Endocrine System   *206*
Drugs That Affect the Reproductive System   *207*
Drugs Used for Infection   *209*

Chapter 27   The Pharmacology of Drug Interactions   **217**

Ways In Which Drugs Can Interact   *217*
Drug Toxicity and Interactions   *219*
Drugs That Affect the Autonomic Nervous System   *222*

Suggested Reading   **226**

**Appendix A Look Alike and Sound Alike Drugs—
Avoiding a Fatal Error**   **227**

Appendix B Pretest with Answers   **231**

**Appendix C Sample Examination and Answer Sheet;
Answers for Scoring**   **249**

Index   **269**

Preface

One of the most rapidly growing fields today is pharmaceutical therapeutics. This rapid growth has created opportunities for a variety of well-trained technical personnel: physician's assistants, medical assistants, nursing assistants, and pharmacy assistants. In fact, one of the most rapidly expanding positions is that of the pharmacy assistant—now called, in most states, the pharmacy technician.

The growing demand for these trained technical personnel is due, in large part, to the rapidly expanding area of drug research and drug discovery. The pharmacist simply does not have enough time to keep up with recent advances in drug therapy and new dosage delivery systems, and counseling patients and physicians, in addition to the other duties such as drug dispensing, ordering, and the record keeping which is required by law. This need for well-qualified technicians to perform sophisticated duties has created the requirement for a standardized examination to ensure that the technicians working within a pharmacy uphold an acceptable level of knowledge and integrity. Thus, a national examination for the certification of pharmacy technicians has been created to replace state certification examinations. The Pharmacy Certification Training Board (PCTB) administers this examination for certification of pharmacy technicians (CPhT). The high standards and increasing difficulty of this examination have created a need for a text which, in addition to being useful for the student of pharmacy technology, will address the main features of the examination, providing information, a comprehensive review, and a basis for understanding the concepts addressed in the examination. *Delmar's Pharmacy Technician Certification Exam Review* was written to fill this need. This text was designed for a twofold purpose: to function as a review for technicians familiar with the material and to serve as a learning tool both for students of pharmacy technology and for technicians who have been trained to perform a limited number of duties (such as within a retail pharmacy). These technicians must now become familiar with broader concepts, such as pharmacology and advanced pharmaceutical calculations, in order to become certified.

The text is written in conversational style, to facilitate understanding of difficult concepts among many levels of readers. Foremost in the text is an examination of the routine procedures in the pharmacy: accepting prescriptions, creating patient profiles, processing and filling prescriptions, and maintaining inventory. This portion of the text covers procedures in both the retail and institutional pharmacy settings, and provides comparisons between them. Special care has been taken to discuss not only the procedures themselves but the reasoning behind the procedures—why are they done in a particular way? This approach is not only necessary to understand work within a pharmacy but is critical to doing well on the certification examination.

A large block of chapters dealing with pharmaceutical calculations has also been provided, which covers a large variety of types of calculations that will appear on the examination. These have been presented in a simple, easy-to-understand manner, designed to take the fear out of math. Topics include not only simple dosage conversions but intravenous calculations, pediatric dosages, compounding, and commercial calculations, as well. All math problems are followed by a section containing the correct answers and a detailed explanation of the reasoning and calculations leading to the correct answer. An entire chapter consisting only of math problems, with answers and worked-out solutions, is included as well.

Among the review material provided, the text contains a pretest, which will assist the reader in prioritizing material to review and study. Each chapter begins with a "Quick Study," a concise summary outline of the material within the chapter, which is designed to accommodate readers at different levels of knowledge. In addition, each chapter contains questions or problems to be worked out, with detailed solutions and answers, which will help the reader understand the thought processes that are crucial to understanding and correctly answering the questions on the examination. Finally, a sample examination is included, with standardized answer sheets, such as those which will be used for the examination.

The author of *Delmar's Pharmacy Technician Certification Exam Review*, Dr. Patricia Anthony, is a practicing pharmacologist with advanced degrees in biology and pharmacology, and bachelor's degrees in biology and pharmaceutical science. In addition, she holds a doctorate in pharmacology from New York Medical College. Before devoting full time to teaching and research, Dr. Anthony devoted full time to medical research as postdoctoral faculty within Harvard Medical School in Massachusetts.

Acknowledgements

The author wishes to thank the reviewers, and especially thanks Mrs. Judie Kautz and Mr. John Carbonaro for their efforts, which made the production of this text possible.

Introduction

About the PCTB Examination

Structure of the Examination

The PCTB examination consists of 125 multiple choice questions. It is a timed test, which lasts for three hours. This means that you must pace yourself in answering the questions. There are three general areas in which competency will be assessed:

1. *Assisting the pharmacist in serving patients.*

   This portion includes interpretation of the prescription order; construction and use of the patient profile; and dispensing, labeling, storage, and delivery of medications. Also included are pharmaceutical calculations: dosage conversions, intravenous medications, IV admixtures, dose per time, and commercial calculations. These questions will make up 50% of the exam (about 60–70 questions). Both hospital and retail settings will be covered, and the student will be expected to know the differences in procedures between the different settings. The questions will require you to think about why you are doing things a certain way as well (with responsibility comes challenge). For example, why is certain information required on the prescription order and profile? Why do we have the patient profile? Why do we use aseptic technique when preparing intravenous medications? This book will train you to think about these things as you answer the questions.

2. *Medication distribution and inventory control.*

   This portion addresses how the medication is stored in the pharmacy, the ordering and inventory process, prepackaging and unit dose distribution, labeling, and record-keeping. These questions will make up 35% of the exam (40–50 questions).

3. *Pharmacy operations.*

This section addresses safety concerns, cleanliness, infection control, pharmacy law, communications, and automation (e.g., computers). These questions make up 15% of the exam.

Taking the Examination

You should read the booklet which came with your application carefully. It contains a lot of useful information, such as the location where the exam will be given and what you should bring with you. You should also be aware that the actual examination will not simply test on memorized information. Questions and problems will require the student to think and synthesize information. It is also helpful if you know how to take the test (see below). When using this text to prepare for the exam, bear in mind that the certification examination is now a national examination, and, since laws vary from state to state, information that may be considered correct for the examination may not be exactly the same as what you have learned in practice.

Answering Questions on the Examination

Since the test is in multiple choice format, you must know how to take multiple-choice tests. You will not know all of the information; however, you can use what you do know to choose the correct answer.

Perhaps a question asks which of the following drugs is a diuretic. The potential answers are: streptomycin, penicillin, tobramycin, and mannitol. You panic, because you have no clue. Instead, you should look carefully at the answers, bearing in mind that only one is correct. Everyone (hopefully) knows that penicillin is an antibiotic. Scratch that one. Two of the answers end in the same thing: strepto*mycin* and tobra*mycin*. It is likely that they do similar things. The only one that is left is mannitol, which happens to be the right answer. If you take the time to look at the question and all of the answers given, before you panic, and think your way through the problem, using the knowledge that you do have, it is time well spent.

Another thing which you must do is to read the question *carefully*. Ask yourself "What is the question asking?" Then, if you can, answer the question in your head before looking at the answers. If you do not, the answers will confuse you. A standard way of making up multiple choice tests is to ask a question and then think of all of the ways a student could interpret the question, or the mistakes which could easily be made, and then make the incorrect answers from that. It is not that the exam is unfair; the questions are simply testing your knowledge and that includes the ability to distinguish fine points. So always answer the question first in your head, and then look for your answer in the choices.

Do not let the questions or answers intimidate you. Let's say you are answering a math problem. You come up with an answer and find it in the list, but the other answers are the same as yours, except for a zero or decimal place. If you did the calculation correctly, your answer is correct. Do not second-guess yourself. More wrong answers are made on exams because students get nervous and change their initial (correct) answer to another (incorrect) answer. You have prepared for this exam—act like it! Have confidence in what you can do.

Don't panic! This exam, like many standardized exams, does not have one passing score. The passing score is different for each exam, because the people who make up the questions assign a difficulty rating to each question, and the average difficulty rating for all of the questions on a particular exam determines the passing score. Thus, the passing score for an exam given in one session will not be the same as another, as the examinations vary in difficulty. Bear this in mind, and if the questions seem to be extremely difficult, don't despair. This may mean that the passing score is lower as well. Just don't panic—just attack the exam logically.

Preparing for the Examination

First, take the "pretest" to determine which sections of the book to review first. There is a "Quick Study" guide at the beginning of each chapter for quick review. Study this first, then read through the chapters for approaches to thinking and important details. Then, as you continue to go through the book, practice doing the problems in each section, even if they seem too easy or hard. The answers are explained for you, so use these to channel your thinking about how to approach the questions in a certain way. Ask yourself questions about the material, and see if you can come up with the answers either on your own or from the text material. Ask *why*! Finally, take the practice test.

When you take the practice test, you will sit in a room with conditions which may not be the best for you. The examination center may not be as warm or as cool as you like, and there will be many other people there who will be making at least a small amount of noise (excessive erasing, drumming fingers or tapping feet, clearing throats, heavy breathing, etc.). I once took a standardized exam next to a student who started with finger drumming, progressed to slapping his feet on the floor, and then [unbelievably] to belching, all simply because he was nervous. Practice concentrating under these conditions—anyone can concentrate in a climate-controlled, comfortable, quiet room! If you can do well under the worst conditions, you will do even better should the conditions be the most favorable for you. If possible, have some others next to you when taking the practice test. These exams are often in close quarters. Finally, grade the exam, using the answer key. Determine which questions you missed and why. Study those parts again.

Now you have prepared for most things which can come your way (one can never be prepared for everything—that's where the thinking part comes in). You are ready to take the exam.

Before the Examination–Helpful Hints

Get a good night's sleep before the exam. Know where the exam is to be held, exactly how to get there, and where to park. Make a dry run, in order to find out how much time it will take you to get there, park, and get to the examination room, then add an extra few minutes This way, when the test day arrives, you will be there on time with a minimum of frustration.

Get adequate nutrition before the exam. Remember—the brain runs on glucose. If you do not feed it, it will not work. So, on the morning of the exam, be sure to eat a good breakfast, even if you are not hungry. This is more important than you might think! Avoid drinking a lot of coffee; substitute juices instead.

You have prepared, so you should not be nervous. If you are, try looking over the section outlines in the book or notes that you have taken for yourself. If it all looks too familiar, you should be ready.

Good luck!

SECTION I

Assisting the Pharmacist in Serving Patients

Chapter 1   Receiving the Medication Order

Chapter 2   Processing the Medication Order

Chapter 3   Preparation and Utilization of the Patient Profile

Chapter 4   Handling Medications

Chapter 5   Proper Storage and Delivery of Drug Products

Chapter 6   Receiving Monetary Compensation for Goods and Services

Receiving the Medication Order

Quick Study

(See text for full explanation.)

I. **Written prescriptions: the prescription blank**

A. **Required information at time of acceptance**—written in ink or typed on the prescription form

- *The patient's full name*
- *Date of issue of the prescription:* regular prescriptions are valid for one year; prescriptions for controlled substances (Schedule II–V) are valid for as little as three days, depending on the state of issue
- *The name and title of the prescriber*
- *The Drug Enforcement Agency (DEA) number* assigned to the prescriber: a seven-digit number, beginning with two letters, denoting the status and last initial of the prescriber
- *The name of the drug* prescribed (generic or brand name)
- *Strength and dosage form* of the drug prescribed (see exceptions)
- *Quantity of drug* to be dispensed
- *Instructions for dosage (SIG)*
- *Instructions for labeling*
- *Signature* of the prescriber, in ink
- *Authorization to dispense a generic substitution*: required for substitution of proprietary label *only*. When "dispense as written" (DAW) designation is present, there is to be no substitution of *any kind*
- *Refill information:*
  1. Must be clearly written in (or the number of refills circled) on the form
  2. *Refill authorization*: an extension of the original prescription. This is the responsibility of the pharmacist
- *Instructions for preparation of the drug*: detailed instructions must be given for preparation; otherwise, it is considered **extemporaneous compounding**, and must be done by the *pharmacist*

B. **Information to be added to the prescription form at time of acceptance**
- *The address and telephone of the patient*: to identify the patient and assist in medication recalls
- *Age or date of birth of the patient*: to identify the patient and clarify proper dose
- *Allergies and concurrent medications*: to prevent potential drug interactions, adverse effects, and therapeutic duplications
- *The insurance coverage of the patient*

C. **Authentication and clarification of the order**
- *Verification of medication* and *amount prescribed, signature* verification
- *Verification of DEA number*

D. **Accepting prescriptions for controlled substances**
- *All information must be present on triplicate form*: no writing on the form is allowed
- *No corrections, writeovers, or extra writing* should ever be present

II. **Prescriptions received by electronic means (telephone, fax machine, or modem)**
- *Accepted by licensed practitioner* (i.e., pharmacist, intern, nurse) *only*
- *Prescription must be immediately transcribed onto a "hard copy"*

III. **Medication Administration Record (MAR)**
A. **Structure and use of the MAR**
- It serves as a drug order in an institutional pharmacy
- It is much more detailed than the paper prescription
- Information presented may include *patient location, billing number, diagnosis, height, weight, medical tests, diet, and medical history*
- Regular medications are ordered by *administration schedule,* according to the twenty-four hour clock
- It may include *directions for use of medications and/or instructions for compounding*
- The organization of the MAR differs from that of the paper prescription
- The *initiation of drug therapy and discontinuation* are specified

B. **Executing the MAR**
- Calculation of the amount of drug required per dose (*unit dose*)
- Preparation of the *correct amount of drug* in the *correct vehicle* for delivery
- Preparation and placement of the *appropriate label*, showing the *patient name, location, drug name, quantity, expiration date, attending physician's name, and instructions* (if any)
- Placement of the prepared unit dose into an appropriately labeled cassette

C. **Comparison of medication orders in retail and institutional settings**
- *Differences in amount of detail presented*: instructions, dosing schedules, etc.

- *More detailed identifying information presented* on the MAR: helps ensure the administration of drugs to the proper patient
- *More information is present* on the MAR: laboratory tests, diet, etc.
- *Concurrent medications are normally not recorded* on the MAR: intake of both food and drugs are more strictly regulated in an institutional setting
- *DEA numbers of individual prescribers are not required*
- *Special documentation for controlled substance prescription is not required on the MAR*

The Medication Order

In a retail pharmacy, the medication order (prescription) is written on a form which is normally preprinted with certain information. If the required information is not preprinted, it may be written or typed on the form. The written medication order must be written in ink or typed, to avoid possible alteration, and must contain the following information when received in the pharmacy. If the prescription is incomplete or illegible it cannot be filled, and the patient should be referred back to the prescriber or to the pharmacist.

Information on the upper portion of the prescription form must include the following:

- **The patient's full name**: This is required for positive identification.
- **The date of issue of the prescription**: The date of writing helps to determine if the prescription may be filled. It should be noted that the laws regarding prescription filling do vary from state to state. However, since the certification exam is based on federal laws, the normal rule of thumb to remember is this: regular prescriptions are valid only for one year after being written, and prescriptions for controlled substances are valid for only three days. If the date of issue is past the date of acceptance (i.e., one year), the prescription cannot be filled.
- **The name and title of the prescriber:** the prescriber may be a doctor of medicine (MD), osteopathic medicine (DO), optometry (OD), dentistry (DDS), veterinary medicine (DVM), or podiatry. Other individuals licensed to prescribe drugs may include the physician's assistant and nurse practitioner.
- **The DEA number of the prescriber**: The DEA number is a seven-digit number issued to the prescriber or institution by the Drug Enforcement Agency. It should begin with two letters. The first letter designates the status of the prescriber (e.g., MD, DO, or nurse practitioner). The second letter is the first letter of the prescriber's last

name. Thus, it is easy to check the validity of the prescription: if the prescriber's name is Smith, for example, and the DEA number starts with AU, it is invalid. A valid DEA number can also be checked by adding the first three odd-numbered digits (the first, third, and fifth numbers) to the sum of the even-numbered digits (the second, fourth, and sixth) multiplied by two. The last digit of this number should be the same as the last digit of the prescriber's DEA number. The authenticity of the prescription can thus be verified by comparing the letters in the DEA number against the name and status of the practitioner, and by numerical calculation.

On the body (middle part) of the prescription you should find all of the following (see Chapter 2 for discussion):

- **The name of the drug prescribed** (generic or brand name).
- **Strength and dosage form** of the drug prescribed (e.g., 10 mg tablets).
- **Quantity of drug to be dispensed** (e.g., 10 tablets, 50 ml).
- **Instructions for dosage (SIG)**: These should be clear and understandable. (See Chapter 2 for a discussion of dosage instruction interpretation.)
- **Instructions for labeling**: The prescriber may not want all of the information on the prescription form to be shown on the label. In this case, instructions as to what information is to be printed on the label are included.
- **Signature of the prescriber, in ink**: no prestamped facsimiles are acceptable.
- **Authorization to dispense a generic substitution**: The way in which generic substitutions are authorized or disallowed varies from state to state. Some states have an open box printed on the prescription form in which the prescriber writes the letters DAW, if the prescription is to be filled exactly as written. In other states, the prescription blank has two lines for signature, and the line on which the prescriber signs designates how the prescription is to be filled (see Chapter 2 for further discussion of generic substitutions).
- **Refill information**: The number of refills should be clearly designated on the prescription form.
- **Instructions for the preparation of a drug**: This is rarely seen on a paper prescription; however, if a drug needs to be made a certain way, such as in a cream or suppository instead of a tablet, the prescriber may write out instructions for preparation of the drug. If specific, written instructions exist for preparation of the drug, it may be prepared by the technician; otherwise it is called **extemporaneous compounding** (see Chapter 21) and must be done by the pharmacist.

There is some information which is necessary for the pharmacy to have, in order to protect the patient (and also to protect the pharmacy from liability). This information may be obtained by the technician and written on the prescription form, if the prescription is for a regular prescription drug. If the prescription is for a Schedule II drug, such as morphine, meperidine (Demerol), or oxycodone (Roxicet), all information must be complete before acceptance at the pharmacy window. There should be no blank spaces, incomplete information, writeovers or corrections of any kind.

Information which may be placed onto a regular prescription form at the time of acceptance includes the following:

- **The patient's address and telephone.**
- **Age or date of birth.**
- **Allergies and concurrent medications.**
- **The insurance coverage of the patient**: How does the patient intend to pay? This might be in cash (self-pay), by co-pay (billing the insurance company directly), or receipt for reimbursement, for example.

Accepting Refill Requests

Refill requests for prescriptions other than Schedule II drugs may be made by the patient. These may be made over the telephone or in person. These requests may be accepted by the technician. Since the original prescription is assigned a number when it is filled, the patient can refer to this number for refill information. The appropriate amount of drug is then deducted from the number of remaining prescription refills, and entered into the patient profile (see Chapter 2). Refills are normally spaced out over an appropriate amount of time; however, they may be given all at one time (at the discretion of the pharmacist) if the patient requests it. Sometimes, when the drug is taken for a long period of time (e.g., anti-seizure drugs and anxiolytics), it is less expensive for the patient to buy larger quantities at one time. Conversely, the patient might not be able to afford the entire quantity of drug prescribed and may be allowed to only purchase part of the prescription at a time. These changes are made at the discretion of the pharmacist, as the pharmacist is legally responsible for all that happens in the pharmacy.

Controlled substances, especially Schedule II drugs, are treated in a very different way. These drugs may be filled by the technician, but any refills (available on Schedule III–V drugs only) must be dispensed within a specific time frame to prevent misuse of the drug. In other words, if a prescription is for three months (two refills are allowed on Schedule III–V drugs), refills may only be filled monthly. No refills may be dispensed on a prescription for a Schedule II drug.

Refill authorizations

Sometimes a patient runs out of a needed medication and has not obtained a new prescription. In this case, the pharmacy may contact the physician/prescriber to extend the original prescription. This is called a refill authorization and may only be obtained by the pharmacist (or pharmacy intern), not the technician. In some states, refill authorizations may be accepted by a technician under the supervision of a pharmacist, but in general this is not the case.

Authentication and Clarification of the Written Medication Order

In the event that the prescription form is unreadable or questionable, the technician should ask the pharmacist for clarification. Often the handwriting of the prescriber is illegible, or the signature or other information is questionable. In this case, the pharmacist will be aware of normal prescribed amounts for the drug in question and will be able to easily clarify the instructions and verify the prescription by telephone with the prescriber. This is especially important in the case of written prescriptions for Schedule II drugs, as they are sometimes altered by the patients in order to use the drug for abuse or sale.

Prescriptions for Schedule II (Controlled Substance Drugs)

The written prescriptions for these drugs must be on a special prescription form. In most states, this is a triplicate form, with the copies of the form serving as records for dispensing: one copy is sent to the Drug Enforcement Agency, one is sent to the prescriber, and one is filed in the pharmacy.

As discussed previously, no information may be written on the triplicate form by the technician; the form must be complete when presented. A pharmacist may alter the dosage form or strength of the drug after consulting with the prescriber (as long as the total amount of drug dispensed stays the same); however, when the technician receives the prescription form, no errors, corrections, or writeovers should be present. If any corrections or extra writing appears on the form, when it is presented, the prescription should not be filled but should be brought to the attention of the pharmacist. This is a serious problem, as patients may alter prescriptions for use or sale.

Receiving Prescriptions by Electronic Means

Prescriptions may actually be communicated to the pharmacy by several means—by the patient (with valid prescription), or by telephone, fax, or modem ("e-mail"). Prescriptions received electronically must be transcribed onto a prescription form ("hard copy") for purposes of documentation. This may only be done by a licensed practitioner (i.e., the pharmacist). Some states grant licensure to pharmacy interns. Here, telephone prescriptions may also be legally taken by a licensed pharmacy intern. The technician may not take prescription orders from electronic devices.

The Medication Administration Record

The medication administration record (MAR) is found only in a hospital or institutional pharmacy and serves as the drug order. It is very detailed, much more so than a paper prescription.

Structure and Use of the MAR

The MAR includes the prescriber's name and title, with the name and age of the patient, like the paper prescription, but also includes other information to identify the patient, such as the hospital identification/billing number assigned to the patient and the patient's location (e.g., [room] 222-[bed number] 1). This helps to prevent delivery of a medication to the wrong patient, and makes billing easier. The information on the MAR may also include the patient's diagnosis, medical history, special diet (if any), and medical tests to be performed on the patient. (If this information is not on the MAR, it will be found on the patient profile [see Chapter 2].)

Unlike the paper prescription, the list of medications ordered for the patient includes a **schedule** for the administration of the drugs, and, if necessary, **instructions for preparation of the drugs**. By looking at the dosage schedule and the age, medical history, diet, and diagnosis of the patient, the pharmacist can doublecheck whether the patient is receiving the appropriate drug for the diagnosis and also whether the drug will aggravate an existing medical condition or interact with food in the patient's diet (see Chapter 27). Medication orders must also specify the **exact dosage form of the drug** (i.e., solution, suspension, tincture, etc., not just "liquid"), strength, and, where appropriate, directions for use. The dosage form ordered should be appropriate to the patient's medical condition; a vomiting patient would not be prescribed an oral medication, for example, but would receive the medication in suppository form or by injection. Again, as in the paper prescription, if there is only one dosage form or strength to the prescribed medication, it is not specified. However, in the hospital setting, the **directions for administration** of the drug must also be specified; an order for morphine gr 1/4 could be given orally, intravenously, or intramuscularly. Since the technician must know how to prepare the drug (size of injection, size of needle, etc.), the **route of administration** must also be specified.

Often, patient medications need to be prepared in a certain way. The MAR may contain **instructions for the proper dilution of a drug** and the **diluent** (the liquid that the drug is to be dissolved in) to be used. Frequently, a patient who is undernourished, vomiting, or has severe diarrhea may require intravenous feeding, and **total parenteral nutrition** solutions (TPNs) may be ordered. These medications contain a balanced mixture of sugars, proteins, and fats to be administered intravenously. The exact mixture depends on the patient's needs, so **instructions for compounding** (how to make the solution) are also stamped or written on the MAR.

The organization of the MAR and instructions for dosage are also very different as compared to the paper prescription. The organization of the MAR varies from hospital to hospital. Some hospitals use a form that lists the **drugs to be administered**, with the **route of administration** (IM, IV, etc.), the **date of order** and **start date of the medication**, and, if warranted, when the drug is to be discontinued (the **duration of therapy** is usually specified with antibiotics or anti-cancer treatments, for example) with the **prescriber name and signature** (authorization), and the **dosage instructions** of each drug all on one line. A checkbox is provided next to the drug name, which the prescriber may use to authorize **generic drug substitution**. The **indication for the use** of the medication (e.g., Lomotil 2.5 mg PO for diarrhea, or Reglan 150 mg IV for nausea, etc.) is also recorded.

Normally, however, instead of giving a set of instructions with each drug (the SIG), the MAR puts the medication orders within a **dosage schedule**. This schedule tells when the drug medications are to be given to the patient and is normally determined by the institution; most hospitals have set times when "routine" medication is delivered, in order to decrease confusion and minimize the possibility of dosage errors. Because this is a hospital the patient will be taking several drugs at a time, on different schedules, as compared to the patient who walks into a pharmacy and has only one drug prescription filled at a time and receives instructions for taking that one drug. In an institution or hospital, drug dosages have to be scheduled relative to each other and are usually administered according to the hospital work shift or during preset medication administration times for the hospital. So, the MAR usually contains a dosage schedule for drug administration. To do this, the MAR lists the times of administration across the top of the page according to a twenty-four-hour clock, with a mark put in the block underneath the time that the medication is to be given to the patient, or places the time by workshift. Next to the time of administration, there may be blank spaces for the technician to note the time of dispensing of the dose and his or her initials and for the nurse to initial as to the time of administration. In this way, an accurate record is kept of when the drug was dispensed and how long the drug was stored before it was given, as well as a record that the drug actually was administered, by whom, and the actual time of administration (this is particularly important with narcotic drugs).

Executing the MAR

To execute ("fill") a MAR, the technician may calculate the amount of drug to be dispensed for each dose, count the proper number of tablets or draw up the injection, and send the dose up to the floor at the proper time in a container properly labeled with the patient's name, patient's hospital number, attending physician's name, and location. However, in reality, single doses are rarely sent up from the pharmacy; rather, the unit dose system is used, in which the drugs are prepared at one time and distributed to the patient floors. The individual drugs are read off of the MAR, with the dosage strength, form, and instructions. The technician is responsible for assessing the instructions for dosage of the drug (e.g., one tablet bid, qid, etc.), and calculating the amount of drug (the number of tablets, number of milliliters, etc.) that will be given to the patient in the course of one day. The technician then prepares the proper amount and places it in a properly labeled container for delivery (cassette). Modern pharmacies now use medication carts, which are located on the individual patient floors. These carts are free-standing, often computerized, cabinets containing the daily medications for all patients on a particular floor or wing within a hospital or nursing home. The technician delivers the unit dose cassettes to the patient floor and files the medications within the drawers of the medication cart, so that enough drug is sent up for an entire day at one time. Normally, the drugs for an individual patient are filed by patient identification number. Unused medication (medication intended for dosing "as needed," for example, and not used, or medication assigned to a discharged patient), if the package has not been opened, may be returned to the pharmacy for re-stocking and patient credit.

Comparison of Medication Orders in Retail and Institutional Settings

The two types of medication orders have many things in common—the name of the patient and other identifying information, the prescriber name and title, and drugs prescribed. The major difference is in the amount of detail presented.

The MAR gives a **detailed schedule of administration**, and times of dispensing and administration are recorded, with the signature or initials of the appropriate person. The retail order gives only instructions to be followed by the patient, because the medication is self-administered.

There is **more identifying information** present on the MAR, to make sure that the medication is administered to the right patient. The amount of information included on the order differs also; the MAR may include not only drug allergies of the patient, but **diagnosis, laboratory tests, height and weight**, and **other information about the patient**. Concurrent medications are normally not listed, because the patient is expected to take only those medications prescribed within the hospital. Thus, the environment is much more controlled. Also, in an institutional setting, the **prescription of controlled substances** does not require a special form; they are just included on the MAR. Since prescribers may use the DEA number assigned to the hospital, there are no prescriber DEA numbers on the MAR (which may also have several prescribers).

In a retail setting, a prescription for a controlled substance (specifically a schedule II, such as Roxicet or Demerol) requires a triplicate form, which must be filed separately from the other prescription forms, with copies sent to the prescriber and DEA. Delivery of the controlled substances to the hospital floor or unit does, however, require special documentation, including signatures of the technician delivering the medication and the head nurse in the patient care area, documenting transfer of the drug (and responsibility for the drug) from the pharmacy to the patient care area.

Questions for Review

1. Which of the following would be found on a MAR, but not a paper prescription?
    1. Patient name
    2. Diagnosis
    3. Dosage schedule
    4. Drug name, strength, and form
    5. Both 2 and 3

2. Which of the following must be present on the written prescription at the time of acceptance?
    1. The prescriber's signature
    2. The exact name, strength, and form of the drug
    3. The age of the patient
    4. All of the above
    5. Both 1 and 2

3. Which of the following may the technician not perform?
    1. Accept refill requests by telephone
    2. Make refill authorizations
    3. Fill prescriptions
    4. Accept prescriptions by electronic means
    5. Both 2 and 4

4. Which of the following is required on a written prescription but not on a hospital MAR?
   1. The generic name of the drug dispensed
   2. The strength of the drug dispensed
   3. The DEA number of the prescriber
   4. The name of the prescriber

5. You receive a prescription written by a Dr. Smith. The DEA number is AU1234567. You should take the following action:
   1. fill the prescription.
   2. call Dr. Smith's office.
   3. alert the pharmacist.
   4. give the prescription back to the patient, as it is invalid.

6. Prescriptions in the pharmacy may be received:
   1. from a patient, directly.
   2. by fax.
   3. by e-mail.
   4. by telephone.
   5. all of the above

7. Prescriptions received by electronic means:
   1. may be filled directly.
   2. may be taken by the technician.
   3. must be transferred to paper (a hard copy) before being filled.
   4. prescriptions are not taken by electronic means.

8. You receive a prescription for secobarbital, which was written two weeks ago. You should:
   1. fill the prescription.
   2. consult the pharmacist.
   3. refuse to fill the prescription and give it back to the patient.
   4. call the prescriber for authorization.

9. You receive a prescription for a drug that is only available by brand name. The prescriber has written the generic name on the prescription. You should:
   1. fill the prescription with the brand-name drug.
   2. consult the pharmacist.
   3. tell the patient that the prescription cannot be filled.
   4. call the prescriber for authorization to dispense the brand-name drug.
   5. Either 1 or 2 would be acceptable.

10. You receive a prescription for Roxicet. You enter the following data on the prescription form:
    1. the address of the patient.
    2. the age of the patient.
    3. the insurance coverage of the patient.
    4. all of the above.
    5. none of the above.

Solutions to Questions for Review

1. The paper prescription contains only the information needed to fill the prescription, dosage directions, and information given by the patient. Therefore, the diagnosis and dosage schedule would not be included; however, they would be found on a MAR. The correct answer is **5**.

2. When the prescription is received, it must contain certain information relating to the patient and prescriber. Information such as the patient's address, age, and allergies may be taken at the time of acceptance. Therefore, the correct answer is **5**, as the age may be added by the technician.

3. The technician may fill prescriptions that have been properly documented (i.e., a hard copy prescription). Since refill requests are made on a previously filled (documented) prescription, and prescriptions are normally filled off of hard copy prescriptions, the technician may do both of these. However, prescriptions submitted by electronic means must be transferred to a hard copy form by the pharmacist (or intern) before filling, and refill authorizations may only be taken by the pharmacist. The correct answer is **5**.

4. The drug information on a MAR is essentially the same as the paper prescription; however, a physician practicing in a hospital will have a DEA number on file or may use the DEA number assigned to the hospital. Therefore, the DEA number is not required. The correct answer is **3**.

5. The DEA number always starts with two letters: one represents the status of the prescriber, and the second is the first letter of the last name. Therefore, since the DEA number starts with AU, and the prescriber's name is Smith, the number is invalid. You should alert the pharmacist. The correct answer is **3**.

6. Receiving a prescription by electronic means includes fax, modem (e-mail), and telephone. The patient may also bring in the prescription, so the correct answer is **5**.

7. All prescriptions dispensed from the pharmacy must be documented. This means that all must have some sort of paper prescription. Thus, prescriptions received over the telephone, by fax, or by modem must be transcribed by the pharmacist (or intern) before filling. The correct answer is **3**.

8. Prescriptions for controlled substances must be filled within three days of writing. Therefore, the prescription is no longer valid, and should the patient need the drug, the pharmacist must call for a refill authorization. The correct answer is **2**.

9. A prescription that is written for a generic drug may always be filled with a proprietary (brand) name. Thus, you may fill the prescription with the brand name; however, the pharmacist may wish to explain the situation to the patient, so either would be acceptable, depending on the pharmacy. The correct answer is **5**.

10. No information is to be added or changed on a prescription for a schedule II drug (Roxicet). Therefore, the correct answer is **5**.

Chapter 2

Processing the Medication Order

Quick Study

(See text for full explanation.)

I. **Basic terminology**

   A. *Dosage form:* solid dosage form (tablet, capsule), semisolid dosage form (cream, suppository), liquid (syrup, tincture, etc.): and specific applications. Use and handling of drugs in suspension

   B. *Dosage strength:* amount of drug per unit prescribed

   C. *Supply dosage:* amount of drug per unit on hand

   D. *Routes of administration:* correct drug preparation for a specific route of administration and reasoning behind procedures used

II. **Interpretation of a written order:** the paper prescription

   A. *Information required on the prescription form,* use of information, and legality issues

   • Regular drugs
   • Narcotics/Schedule II controlled substances

   B. *Instructions for dosing:* drug doses and half life

   C. *Information to be entered on the form at time of dispensing:* use of information (why is it needed?) and legality issues

   • Indentifying information
   • Age and gender
   • Concurrent medications

   D. *Interpretation of abbreviations* (see text)

   E. Choosing and dispensing the appropriate drug in a correct manner

Basic Terminology—The Dosage Form and Instructions

To correctly process a written medication order, it is necessary to know some basic terminology. When the drug is prescribed, it is usually prescribed in a specific dosage **form**. The form in which the drug is used depends on the condition of the patient; most drugs are taken in tablet form orally (by mouth), but others must be used in a suppository form (e.g., for a vomiting patient), topically, on the skin (for a rash or skin condition), or in liquid form (for a child). Since different dosage forms are packaged and used differently, it is important to know which dosage form the drug must be in. In addition, the instructions written by the prescriber are abbreviated, and the technician must be familiar with these abbreviations to accurately convey the instructions to the patient. (See Table 2–1.)

Solid Dosage Forms

Solid dosage forms are those that can be picked up and handled. These include the oral dosage forms of **tablet**, **capsule**, and **enteric coated tablet**.

A tablet is made of pressed powder. How hard the powder is pressed determines how the tablet can be used. For example, a **sublingual tablet** is made to dissolve quickly, under the tongue, and therefore cannot be pressed hard into a dense tablet. (Since the tablet is so soft, it must be handled very carefully to avoid turning the tablet into a pile of powder.) An example of a sublingual tablet would be a nitroglycerin tablet, which is made to dissolve quickly and be absorbed quickly into the system. A capsule is a gelatin "container" filled with powdered drug, drug granules, a liquid formulation, or an oil. Examples would be a vitamin such as A, D, or E, and many over-the-counter cold remedies.

Liquid Dosage Forms

The liquid dosage forms for oral use include the **syrup**, which is a sweetened liquid, containing the drug and flavoring, and the **elixir**, which is similar to a syrup but contains a relatively high percentage of alcohol. An **extract** is the oil or active portion of a plant or herb, which is usually removed, or extracted, with alcohol. An example might be an extraction of peppermint or wintergreen.

Another oral dosage form is the drug **suspension**, composed of water and drug particles which do not dissolve but remain *suspended* in the water. If the drug dissolves into the liquid, it is called a **solution**. In a suspension, the drug does not dissolve, but simply floats suspended in the water. Suspensions need to be handled carefully, as the drug particles tend to sink to the bottom very quickly. Mixing and drawing the dose can be tricky.

With a suspension, the withdrawal of the drug dose must be done immediately after mixing, before the drug particles have a chance to settle. If the suspension is not properly mixed or the dose is not drawn immediately the wrong dose of drug may be dispensed. If the dose is taken from the top of the container, it may contain too much water; if it is taken from the bottom, the drug solution may be too concentrated because the drug particles tend to sink. In addition to mixing the suspension thoroughly, how the dose is withdrawn matters, as well. In a suspension, the drug particles may sink to the bottom very quickly; so, the dose must be drawn up quickly, as the drug particles may settle while the dose is being drawn.

The **tincture** is another liquid dosage form but, in modern times, is only used topically. The tincture is an alcohol-based drug form, such as tincture of merthiolate, and is normally dispensed in a dropper bottle. These drugs are not to be taken internally.

Semisolid Dosage Forms

The **semisolid** dosage forms include creams, lotions, and ointments. Creams and lotions are nothing more than emulsions—oil droplets suspended in water, where the drug is usually dissolved in the oil. Creams are thicker, as they contain less water than lotions. Ointments may vary from a thick emulsion to a drug suspended in a waxy base, like petrolatum (which is like petroleum jelly, only much stiffer and thicker). These preparations are usually used topically (on the skin or mucous membranes such as those of the mouth, inside of the nose, or rectum) and are normally dispensed in a tube or jar.

Care must be taken in storing emulsions. Freezing the emulsion or exposing it to excessive heat (near a heat source, for example, or storage in a warm room for a long time) will cause the cream to separate into oil and water. Emulsions should not be stored in the refrigerator and especially should never be frozen, as the rapid change in temperature will cause the product to separate faster.

Routes of Administration

The route of administration defines how the drug gets into the body. Drugs to be administered by different routes are prepared in different ways. The most common route of administration is by mouth (P.O.). These drugs are given as a tablet or oral solution. **Sublingual** tablets (SL) are made to dissolve under the tongue (sublingual preparations may also be marketed in a spray formulation), as the underside of the tongue and the floor of the mouth contain large amounts of blood vessels near the surface, which allow the drug to be absorbed into the system very quickly. These tablets are very soft and dissolve easily. Drugs for the eye or ear are administered by drop (gtt). The dropper or dropper container is calibrated to give a drop of the particular size needed to give an accurate dose of drug.

Injections vary according to type. Intravenous injections are prepared in three ways: the **bolus**, which means a one-time injection from a syringe; the **IV drip**, which means a bag or bottle of liquid, which allows drug to be infused over a longer time; and the **"piggyback" IV**, which is a solution contained in a smaller IV bag that is infused into or with the primary intravenous drip.

Intramuscular injections are placed into skeletal muscle. This allows the drug to enter the bloodstream more slowly. These injections require a large bore needle in order to penetrate the muscle.

Injections into or under the skin include subcutaneous (SC) injections and intradermal (ID) injections. SC injections are placed under the skin, which allows for a slow distribution of drug through the body. Intradermal (ID) injections which are less common are placed within the skin layers. These injections must be dispensed with a very fine needle (25-30 gauge) on the syringe.

Intrathecal and **intracardiac** injections are specialized injection forms. Intrathecal injections are placed into the space between the spinal cord and spinal meninges (e.g., an epidural anesthetic during childbirth), and intracardiac injections are placed directly into the heart. These types of injections allow fast action of a drug on a particular organ by placing the drug within the organ itself.

Interpreting the Order

Before filling the prescription, one must first check the prescription form to make sure that the prescription is genuine, legal, and complete, as discussed in Chapter 1. Certain information must be on the prescription form when it is received, and other information may be filled in by the technician, unless the prescription is for a controlled substance, written on a triplicate form. In this case, no information is to be added, deleted, or corrected on the prescription form.

Table 2–1 lists abbreviations commonly used in the information provided on the prescription form by the prescriber. These abbreviations must be interpreted accurately to ensure that the correct medication is dispensed and that accurate instructions are provided to the patient for the use of the medication.

Table 2–1   Abbreviations used on prescription forms

When		Where	
cc	with meals	po	by mouth
ac	before meals (think of a.m.)	od	right eye
		os	left eye
pc	after meals (think of p.m.)	ou	both eyes
		ad	right ear
hs	at bedtime (before sleep)	as	left ear
		au	both ears
qd	once a day (or every day)	IM	intramuscularly
		IV	into the vein: bolus or drip
bid	twice a day	SC	under the skin
tid	three times a day	ID	into the skin
qid	four times a day	IA	into the artery
qod	every other day	IT	intrathecal
q wk	once a week	IC	intracardiac
prn	as needed	SL	sublingual (under the tongue)
ut dict	as directed	rect	rectally, in the rectum
atc	around the clock		
qh	every hour		
c̄	with		
s̄	without		

How much		Drug form	
cc	cubic centimeter (same as ml)	tab	tablet
		cap	capsule
fl	fluid	pul	pulvule
g	gram	syr	syrup
gr	grain	susp	suspension
gtt	drop	el	elixir
mg	milligram	ext	extract
mcg	microgram (μg)	tinct	tincture
aa	of each	ung	ointment
tsp	teaspoon		
T	tablespoon		

It should be noted that these abbreviations may appear in either upper or lower case lettering, depending on the prescriber (most prescribers use lower case letters). Since they are abbreviations, periods may also appear after the letters; however, few prescribers take the time to attend to such details, so periods have been omitted here as well. You may see either upper or lower case lettering (or a combination) on the exam—there is no special meaning attached to capitalization in this case.

Figure 2–1 represents the normal paper prescription that would be received at the pharmacy window. Information required to correctly fill

John Smith M.D.
201 Tablet Lane
Anywhere USA
DEA#AS 1234567

Date _2/1/98_

Name _Sally Swollen_

Address _____

SIG: _Lasix 40mg tabs #60_

℞ _bid prn Edema_

John Smith M.D.

_____   _____
Dispense as Written   May Substitute

Refill   0   1   2   3   4   5

Figure 2–1   Sample completed prescription form

this order is found on the body of the prescription. Review the information required to appear on the prescription:

- **The drug name.** This can be generic (the actual name of the drug substance) or a brand (proprietary) name. This prescription specifies the exact drug to select for dispensing. This prescription was written for a brand name, Lasix.

- **The strength and dosage form of the drug**: Drugs come in different strengths and forms for different needs. The strength and form must be specified unless the drug only comes in one strength (such as a combination drug—Tylenol # 3, for example) or one form (e.g., mannitol injection). Lasix tablets come in 20 mg, 40 mg, and 80 mg strengths, as well as oral solution and solution for injection, so the dosage strength and form *did* need to be specified in this case.

- **The amount of drug** prescribed: Since the prescription in Figure 2–1 is for tablets, the number of tablets to be dispensed was specified. For a liquid dosage form, there is often more than one way that the dosage can be specified. Either the volume may be specified, or the drug dose may be specified in mg, g, and so on. In this case, the volume to be dispensed would have to be calculated.

- **Instructions for the patient** (the SIG): This is where a knowledge of the abbreviations in Table 2–1 comes in. Since the instructions must be written out for the patient, the technician must be able to accurately read the SIG. The prescription in Figure 2–1 states that one tablet (designated by a horizontal bar with one vertical bar and one dot) is to be taken twice a day (bid, or bis in deum), as needed (prn) for edema. The amount of medication to be taken, and when or how often it is to be taken, must be included on the prescription form. The spacing of the doses, or dosage interval, is extremely important, as the space between doses is based on the half-life ($t_{1/2}$) of the drug. Every drug behaves differently in the body; some stay in the body a long time, whereas some are cleared very rapidly. The half-life ($t_{1/2}$) is a measure of how fast the drug is cleared from the body. This number tells us how long it takes for half of the dose to leave the body, or become inactive. A drug with a $t_{1/2}$ of two hours, for example, would be half gone in two hours, half of that would be gone in another two hours (resulting in 3/4 of the original dose gone in four hours), and so on. To keep the level of the drug in the blood as constant as possible for maximum effectiveness, the drug should be replenished as it is cleared. Therefore, accurate, clear dosage instructions are very important. It is also important to communicate clearly to the patient what is to be done with the drug. A tablet would be taken, a suppository would be inserted, an opthalmic preparation would be instilled (placed) in the eye, and so on.

- **Signature of the prescriber and authorization to substitute**: The signature must be handwritten *in ink*. Depending on the state the prescription is written in, there may be one blank for the signature or two. If there are two, the line on which the prescriber signs tells the pharmacy which drugs may be dispensed. The "may substitute" line gives the patient and pharmacy the freedom to choose a cheaper drug, such as a generic form, or have the prescription filled with a different brand name, as long as the drug, strength, and form remain the same. If the signature appears over the "dispense as written" blank (or, in some states, where only one signature line is present, the prescriber writes "DAW" in a box on the prescription form), the exact drug prescribed must be dispensed. There is no freedom on the part of the patient or technician to exchange one brand name for another without the consent of the prescriber (which would have to be obtained by the pharmacist). Dispense as written means exactly that—dispense exactly the drug, form, and proprietary label perescribed. This does not apply to a prescription for a generic drug; however, if the prescription is for a generic drug, the patient may request to have the prescription filled with a generic, or any brand-name of the drug, regardless of the signature line.

- **Refills:** The refill designation may appear as a number circled on the bottom of the regular prescription, or as a number written in a blank which designates refills. If no number is circled or written in, no refills are authorized. No refills may be authorized at any time on a Schedule II drug, and only one refill may be authorized on drugs which fall within Schedules III or IV. On a regular prescription, the technician may legally refill prescriptions only up to the specified number of refills. If the patient requires more medication, he or she must then obtain a new prescription. In an urgent situation (the medication is needed immediately, and there is no time to obtain a new prescription) the pharmacist may call in a **refill authorization** to the prescriber, to extend the prescription. This can only be done by the *pharmacist* (or in some states, a pharmacy intern)—it cannot be done by the technician.

Information to be entered on the prescription form and patient profile by the technician includes the following:

- **The patient's address and telephone**: This information helps to identify the patient should there be more than one patient with the same name. It also serves as a way to contact the patient should there be a problem with a prescription, such as a drug recall or an incorrect drug dispensed.

- **The age or date of birth of the patient**: This information may be useful in two ways. First, age may serve as identifying information. For example, the pharmacy may have a father and son, both patients with the same name, living at the same address. The age would distinguish the two. Second, the age of the patient is also very important in determining whether the drug in the dosage prescribed is appropriate for the patient. Not all patients are alike. As we get older, body functions begin to slow down. The kidney and liver do not work as well, and they may be less effective in clearing the drug from the body. So the drug dose may have to be adjusted in an older patient (see Chapter 27). Some drugs would be much more toxic to an older person than to a twenty-year-old, for example. In the same way, since the organ systems of an infant or small child are still developing, drug doses and choices of therapy would be different for a very young person as well.

- **Drug allergies**: many drugs are very similar in chemical structure and action. Thus, if a patient is allergic to one drug, penicillin, he or she may well be allergic to similar drugs, such as amoxicillin or even cephalexin. A history of drug allergies may help prevent an uncomfortable or even fatal allergic reaction.

- **Concurrent medications**: These are medications already being taken by the patient. Many drugs interact with each other to produce negative side effects, or one drug may dramatically increase or decrease the effect of another (see Chapter 27). A history of concurrent medications should include not only other prescription medications but also those purchased over the counter (e.g., cold remedies), and herbal remedies as well. (Most people do not realize that the first drugs were little more than ground up plants, or plant extracts. We have done little more than refine them, in many cases.) Herbal preparations can have very potent drug actions and interactions and must be recorded in the patient profile.

Dispensing the Correct Medication

Once the drug, dosage form, and strength have been established, the correct medication is selected. This medication should be exactly what appears on the prescription form. Many drug names look alike and sound alike, so the drug labels must be compared carefully to the order. If extra letters are present in the drug name (e.g., Adalat CC instead of Adalat), the drug may be a different formulation of the brand name drug (in this case an extended release form) or a different drug altogether (e.g., quinine and quinidine). If the name of the drug does not match exactly, the drug may not be dispensed (see Appendix A for a list of look-alike and sound-alike drugs). The dosage strength is less critical. If the dosage strength does not match, it may be possible to convert dosages (see Chapters 4 and 14). If the dosage form is incorrect, the drug cannot be dispensed by the technician.

Comparison of Drug Dispensing in Retail and Institutional Settings

Dispensing a prescription in an institutional setting is similar to the retail setting, with a few exceptions. Several drugs are usually prescribed at once (see Chapter 1) using the MAR, and these doses may be sent up to the patient individually (e.g., a medication needed quickly, for an emergency [STAT], or a medication prescribed for pain, emesis, etc., which is not part of the usual routine of drugs) or as a package of drugs that is enough of a particular drug for one day. This package is called a **unit dose**. It is calculated for each drug prescribed by multiplying the frequency of dosing (bid, tid, etc.) by the dose (e.g., 1 tablet). Thus, enough doses to last for the whole day may be sent at one time. Exceptions to unit dosing include medications like creams, lotions, syrups, and topical liquids. Here, instead of calculating how much cream or syrup the patient is to use per day and finding a way to get it to the patient without making a huge mess, we simply dispense an entire tube or bottle of the medication and replace it as needed. Narcotics prescribed "as needed" may not be dispensed in a unit dose.

Questions for Review

1. You receive a shipment of lotion that appears to have separated into two layers, within the bottle. The shipment has probably:
   1. always been this way.
   2. been exposed to extreme heat.
   3. been frozen and allowed to thaw out, perhaps more than once.
   4. either 2 or 3 could be correct.

2. A prescription for a Timoptic reads "1 gtt ou bid." The instructions would be:
   1. take one drop twice a day.
   2. take 1 ml twice a day.
   3. insert one drop in each ear twice a day.
   4. place one drop in each eye twice a day.

3. In an institutional setting, a prescription for Lasix would be:
   1. automatically filled generically.
   2. filled with Lasix only.
   3. filled with any similar brand name diuretic, if the pharmacy is out of Lasix.
   4. filled with Lasix unless the prescriber has indicated on the MAR that a substitution is permissible.

4. Which of the following is not a solid dosage form?
   1. Capsule
   2. Pulvule
   3. Cream
   4. Tablet

5. In an institutional setting, medications are normally filled:
   1. by unit dose.
   2. by individual dose.
   3. in bulk, so that the nurses can help themselves.
   4. by paper prescription.

6. You receive a prescription for Procardia, ordered "Dispense as Written." You check the stock and find Procardia XL. You:
   1. fill the prescription with the available stock.
   2. fill the prescription, but adjust the dosage according to the label on the bottle.
   3. tell the patient that the prescription cannot be filled.
   4. fill the prescription with Adalat, as it is the same thing.

Solutions to Questions for Review

1. Emulsions, such as lotions, are delicate mixtures of oil and water. Rapid changes in temperature or prolonged exposure to very hot or cold temperatures will cause them to separate. The correct answer is **4.**

2. Even if you don't remember the notations, your first clue should be the brand name, Tim*optic*; gtt = drop, o = eye, u = both, bid means two times a day. Since the medication is to be placed into the eye, the correct answer is **4**.

3. The MAR normally contains a space for the prescriber to indicate whether substitution is authorized. Occasionally, if the name-brand drugs are too expensive or will not be covered by insurance, an institution may dictate that only generics will be dispensed, but usually, substitutions occur because the pharmacy simply does not stock the name-brand drugs. Generally, if a prescriber orders a name-brand drug, it must be dispensed accordingly. The correct answer is **4**, because the prescriber is given the option to allow generic substitution.

4. Solid dosage forms are, in general, those which can be picked up and handled. The only one that cannot be safely handled is **3**, a cream.

5. Most doses to the patient are dispensed in unit doses. Occasionally, individual doses may be ordered, under special circumstances, but normal dosing is done by **(1)** unit dose.

6. Procardia and Procardia XL (the extended-release form) are not the same. Even though the names look similar, the technician could not dispense this drug for Procardia. The correct answer is **3**, as the prescription cannot be filled.

Chapter 3

Preparation and Utilization of the Patient Profile

Quick Study

(See text for full explanation.)

I. **Obtaining and entering patient information**

   A. Types of information required for patient profile

   B. Patient interview

   C. Updating patient profiles with information regarding new allergies, concurrent medications, change of address, etc.

II. **Purpose and utilization of the patient profile**

   A. *Identification of the patient*

   B. *Serves as a record of medications dispensed to the patient*

   C. *Protects the patient against drugs or procedures that could potentially be harmful*

III. **Organization of the patient profile**

   A. *Identifying information*: name, date of birth, contact information, and insurance information

   B. *Drugs prescribed*: helps to identify potential drug interactions, as new drugs are prescribed

   C. *Drug allergies and adverse reactions*: helps to protect the patient against misprescribed drugs

   D. *Concurrent medications*: helps to prevent drug interactions and therapeutic duplication

   E. *Medical history*: helps to prevent potentially lethal aggravation of existing conditions by prescribed drugs

   F. *Mental conditions, handicaps*: helps to predict the degree of supervision needed with the drug therapy. Physical handicaps such as arthritis may dictate the need for a special cap on the dispensing bottle, or poor eye sight may require large-print labeling and so forth.

G. *Insurance information*

H. *Height, weight, diagnosis, therapies, laboratory tests, and results* (institutional profile): height and weight may be required to calculate accurate drug dosage. Also, hospital patients may need to be weighed to determine weight loss or gain. Diagnosis, concurrent therapies, and test results may help the pharmacist check for accurate therapeutic prescribing.

IV. **Comparison of the patient profile in the institutional and retail settings**

A. *More details are included in the institutional setting*: goals of therapy, special diet, diagnosis, tests, billing information, billing number, etc.

B. *Slight differences in the type of information included*: refill information and concurrent medications are not applicable to the institutional profile

Obtaining and Entering Patient Information

The patient profile is a means of distinguishing and identifying patients, serves as a record of medications dispensed, and, most importantly, is a resource of information that could protect the patient against potentially harmful drugs or procedures. The profiles in an outpatient and institutional setting contain similar information; however, the information contained in a patient profile within an institutional setting (e.g., hospital or nursing home) tends to be more detailed. The following are included in an outpatient profile:

- Identifying information: This includes the patient's name, address, telephone, and date of birth.

- Drug allergies and adverse reactions (negative effects, caused by a drug): many times, when a patient is allergic or sensitive to one type of drug, the allergy will extend to similar drugs as well. Rarely, food allergies will cause problems in the tolerance of a drug due to the drug "carrier" which is what the drug is put into in order to give it enough volume to swallow or inject.

- Use of more than one medication at the same time (concurrent medications): Many drugs interact with each other. They may produce similar effects which will be additive with each other, they may amplify each other's effects (synergism), or they may reduce the effectiveness of each other (antagonism). This may happen in different ways (see Chapter 27). The use of one drug at the same time as another may, because of storage within the body, increase the blood levels of the other drug, requiring a change in the dosage of the drug(s). Concurrent medications are very important, and, because drugs sold over-the-counter are the same (or similar) to those sold by prescription, *all* medications taken, including herbal preparations, must be recorded.

Another reason that we need to determine concurrent patient medication is to see if any of the drugs prescribed are the same (**drug duplication**). If two prescriptions contain the same drugs, under different names, one must be eliminated. Possibly, the patient has been prescribed a drug by one prescriber, and has also received a prescription for a combination drug from a second prescriber which contains the same drug (or is the same drug under a different brand name). This applies to the over-the-counter medications as well, which may contain lower amounts of various prescription drugs.

- Medical history: This includes any medical conditions which the patient may have and may also include the patient's immediate family. Certain medical conditions will be aggravated by certain drugs, which should be avoided. If the patient's family members have inherited medical conditions that have not yet developed in the patient, it is reasonable to assume that these conditions could develop at any time, and the possibility exists that certain drugs or procedures could be harmful, even though the condition has not yet developed.

- History of mental problems or drug abuse: This may indicate that the patient is not competent to use the medication properly. In an outpatient setting, this may mean that the patient must be supervised more closely and that the amount of medication given out at one time may be more strictly regulated.

- Special considerations: Any physical, mental, or cultural handicaps should be addressed. For instance, whether a patient is handicapped in any way. A patient with limited vision may need large-print labels on the dispensing container and another with a hearing deficit may need special attention during drug counseling by the pharmacist. A person with arthritis may need to have easy-open caps on dispensing bottles. Also, patients from other cultures may need special consideration due to language or to cultural and religious beliefs.

- Insurance information: This includes determination of insurance eligibility, the type of third-party payment (co-pay or self pay, etc.), and the coverage of prescribed drugs. Insurance coverage varies widely among the various insurance plans. Many plans will no longer pay for certain drugs, due to price. Some will authorize only payment for generic drugs, and others will authorize payment for proprietary label drugs only under certain circumstances (i.e., if no other drug is available or the drug is needed for a life-threatening condition).

- Current prescriptions and refill information: The outpatient profile will show the status of the patient's various prescriptions, so that the amount dispensed and the amount available on the prescription remain current. This needs to be updated with each prescription refill.

The institutional patient profile may also include the patient's height, weight, diagnosis, treatment, therapy, diet plans, blood tests, and lab results, as well as the name of the primary physician. However, the institutional profile would not include information which is not applicable to institutional policy, such as refill information and concurrent medications other than those prescribed within the institution.

The technician creates a profile for every patient receiving medications from the pharmacy. Normally, the format for the profile is contained in the pharmacy computer program, and the information is entered into the program. Patients who are new to the pharmacy must be interviewed to obtain the information that is necessary for creation of the profile.

Where patients have existing profiles (repeat patients), the profiles just need to be updated with each visit. If any information has changed, such as allergies, concurrent medications, insurance information, or address and telephone, for example, this information needs to be changed in the profile to reflect the correct information. This may require an additional patient interview if the changes are lengthy; the patient must at least be asked if the personal information is current and if he or she is taking any new drugs or has experienced any problems with the medication. In addition, the pharmacist may require that the patient be asked about changes in his or her medical condition. The reason for updating the patient profile is to make sure the pharmacist has the most recent information to take into consideration when counseling the patient, so that appropriate advice will be given.

Comparison of Patient Profiles in Institutional and Retail Settings

In general, the profiles in the institutional setting are more detailed than those in the retail or outpatient setting. Profiles in both settings contain information used to locate and identify the patient (address and phone in the retail or outpatient setting, and room and bed number in the institutional setting), insurance information, date of birth, and medications prescribed. In addition, profiles in both settings include the prescriber's name and the date that the medication was prescribed and dispensed. In the institutional setting, the profile also includes the date and time of day that the medication was prescribed and dispensed, billing information, and more detailed information such as diagnosis, therapeutic goals, and diagnostic tests.

Some major differences between the profiles in the retail and institutional settings include the following:

- Institutional (hospital) profiles may include diagnosis, a statement of the goals of the therapy, special diet (if any), medical tests that the patient has undergone, and the results of those tests. Since the profile may serve as a document for billing the patient, billing information may also be included as well as prices of the medication. Also included is the hospital billing number assigned to the patient, which gives the billing department access to all insurance information.

- Retail pharmacy profiles do not contain this information. However, since the patient may be taking many drugs concurrently, the retail profile does contain a list of concurrent medications. This is not the case in the hospital profile, as drugs of any kind are discouraged, other than those dispensed by the hospital pharmacy. Refill information is included in an outpatient (retail pharmacy) profile but would not be appropriate in a hospital or institutional profile.

Questions for Review

1. The following would be found on a patient profile, under "concurrent medications:"
   1. prescription drugs
   2. nonprescription drugs, such as Tylenol and aspirin
   3. herbal medications such as herbal diuretics and golden seal
   4. all of the above

2. A patient profile would be created for:
   1. a hospital inpatient.
   2. a new patient to a pharmacy.
   3. a regular pharmacy customer.
   4. anyone who receives prescription medications from any pharmacy.

3. A former patient comes to the pharmacy with a prescription. His address has changed. You should:
   1. take the new information and update his patient profile.
   2. advise the pharmacist.
   3. put him in as a new patient and create a new profile.
   4. ignore the information, as the address is not important.

4. The patient in question #3 comes back with a new prescription and has a rash from the pre-scription that he had filled a few days ago. You should:
   1. note the rash in the "allergies" section of his patient profile.
   2. alert the pharmacist.
   3. fill the new prescription.
   4. ignore the rash, as it is minor.

5. The following would be found on a patient profile in the retail setting but not the hospital setting:
   1. patient identification
   2. diagnosis and lab test results
   3. concurrent medications
   4. drug allergies

6. An example of a medication duplication would be:
   1. a prescription for trimethoprim and another for sulfisoxazole.
   2. a prescription for Tylenol #3, and the patient is taking acetominophen capsules.
   3. a prescription for generic digoxin and for Digibind.
   4. a prescription for an antihistamine given to a patient taking aspirin.
   5. both 2 & 3

Solutions to Questions for Review

1. Concurrent medications are those which the patient is taking at the same time as the prescription drug. These include any medications, whether they are over-the-counter drugs such as aspirin; prescription drugs; or potent herbal medications, such as "herbal Fen-Fen" or golden seal, both of which mimic the sympathetic nervous system and act as sympathomimetic drugs. The correct answer is **4**.

2. A patient profile must be created for *anyone* receiving prescription drugs from a pharmacy. The correct answer is **4**.

3. A change in demographic information (address, phone) must be recorded in the profile but is not of sufficient importance to report to the pharmacist. The technician may simply update the profile. The correct answer is **1**.

4. An important change in the reported information on a patient, such as the development of a rash, could be a symptom of a serious drug allergy. The pharmacist should be alerted. The correct answer is **2**.

5. The question asks what would be found in the retail setting; those are—**1 and 3**. Now, the question asks which of these would not be found on a hospital profile. Patient identification would be found on both, so the correct answer is **3**, concurrent medications.

6. A medication duplication means two of the same drug, or drugs which do exactly the same thing. Trimethoprim and sulfisoxazole are both antibiotics but may be used together. Antihistamines and aspirin are not related, so that leaves **2 & 3**. Tylenol #3 contains acetominophen, so it would be a duplication to take acetominophen as well. The correct answer is **2**.

Chapter 4

Handling Medications

Quick Study

(See text for full explanation.)

I. **Obtaining the correct medication from inventory**
   A. Interpretation of the manufacturer's label
   B. Dosage conversions

II. **Proper dispensing procedures for various dosage forms**
   A. Solid, liquid and semi-solid dosage forms
   B. Appropriate dispensing containers
   C. Proper labeling procedures
   - *Information required* on the label
   - Proper tabulation of *prescriber's instructions*
   - Use of *auxiliary labels*
   D. Bulk compounding and bulk manufacturing
   E. Preparation of sterile solutions
   - Aseptic techniques and why they are used
   - Proper use of a laminar flow hood

III. **Preparation of parenteral injections**
   A. *Subcutaneous* injections
   B. *Intramuscular* injections
   C. *Intravenous* injections
   - Bolus
   - Large volume injectables

IV. **Preparation of admixtures**
   A. "Piggyback" IV's
   B. Mixing admixtures
   C. Proper labeling of injections and admixtures

Use of the Manufacturer's Label to Correctly Dispense Medication

After the prescription form has been received and processed, the next step is to obtain the correct medication from inventory. When selecting the medication, one must look closely at the manufacturer's label. Is the name of the drug, the strength, the form, and the manufacturer of the drug exactly the same as what was ordered? All of the information on the drug label must match the order, with the exception of the dosage strength. If the dosage strength is not appropriate for the order, calculations may be done to determine if the dosage strength can be converted to what is needed. Let's say that the order asks for a dose of 100 mg po, and the tablets in stock are 200 mg. If the tablets are scored (a groove runs across the tablet) so that we can accurately break them in half, we can put instructions on the label for the patient to take one-half tablet per dose (100 mg). This is called **dosage conversion** (see Chapters 14 and 15) and is perfectly acceptable as long as the calculated dose is accurate. We cannot do this with everything. If the tablet is scored in half, we can fill the order by breaking the tablets at the groove. However, if it is scored in thirds (Ⓨ) or not scored at all, we cannot accurately determine what portion of the tablet is 100 mg, and cannot fill the order.

Liquid medications are handled a little differently. Figure 4–1 shows a label for Vistaril, an oral suspension. The concentration of drug in the suspension is clearly stated on this label, beneath the generic name of the product. The position on the label where the drug concentration is stated may vary from label to label, but it is usually included. If not, it can be easily calculated from the information given (see Chapter 15). We use the

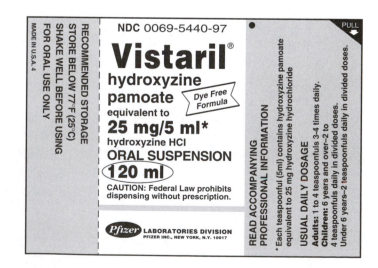

Figure 4-1   Drug label

drug concentration to calculate the proper amount of suspension to dispense for the dosage ordered (see Chapter 15), so an order for almost any dosage can be filled, as long as the amount dispensed is appropriate.

If the information on the manufacturer's label exactly matches the order and the proper dosage can be dispensed, we are ready to measure the drug for dispensing. The solid dosage forms are easy to accurately dispense: we simply count out the tablets, in a sanitary, accurate manner. Liquids, however, must be measured out using properly calibrated equipment and correct procedures (see below).

Packaging and Labeling the Medication

Once the drug has been accurately measured, it should be placed into the proper container and labeled. Containers vary according to the intended use of the drug. For a topical solution, the drug should be placed into a bottle with a dropper cap. If it is a cream or ointment, it should be placed in an ointment tube or jar. A liquid for oral dosing should be placed into an appropriate bottle, usually with a small neck, suitable for slow pouring. Solid dosage forms are placed into large-mouthed dispensing bottles. All dispensing bottles should be sealed with child-proof caps, according to the Poison Prevention and Packaging Act. An "easy-open" cap may be placed on the bottle if the patient signs a waiver form indicating that this type of cap is requested. This releases the pharmacy from liability should accidental poisoning occur due to unsecured packaging.

Care must also be taken to ensure that the size of the dispensing container is appropriate for the amount of medication being dispensed. A container that is too large will allow the medication too much freedom to move, which may result in damage to solid dosage forms. In addition, the general appearance would be sloppy and the patient may have trouble retrieving the medication from the container. A container that is too small may crush tablets or force a liquid or cream out.

Properly Labeling the Container

Once the drug has been packaged, it must be labeled appropriately. Information required to be on a label (unless omissions are requested by the prescriber) is as follows:

- The name, address, and phone of the pharmacy (usually preprinted on the label).
- The name of the patient for whom the drug is intended (or the name of the owner, if the drug is for an animal).
- The name of the prescriber.

- Date of dispensing.
- The name of the drug that was actually dispensed: If the prescription was for a proprietary label (name brand) and the generic was dispensed, the generic name should appear on the label (the manufacturer of the generic drug is usually stated as well). For example, if the prescription was for furosemide, and Lasix was dispensed, the brand-name "Lasix" would appear on the label. If the prescriber requests it, this information may be left off of the label entirely.
- The strength of the medication (40 mg tabs, 5%, etc.). If the drug is only available in one strength or is a combination drug, this may not appear on the label.
- The quantity of drug dispensed (number of tablets, number of milliliters, etc.).
- Directions for use: These should be clear, understandable, and appropriate to the user. For example, if the prescription is for a child, the label should read "Give...[the drug]"; if the drug is for oral dosage, instructions would be "Take..."; for rectal or vaginal use, instructions would be "Insert," and so on.
- Additionally, the label may contain refill information, and usually the initials of the person dispensing the drug will appear by the date of filling.

Dispensing Liquid Medications

We normally dispense liquids differently for different uses. For opthalmic use or use in the ear, drug solutions are usually prepackaged in a sterile bottle with dropper tip. For topical use, solutions are packaged in a dropper bottle (with a dropper in the cap). The majority of liquids, however, are dispensed for either oral use (by mouth) or parenteral use (by injection). An institutional pharmacy would dispense liquids for either oral or parenteral use, while a retail pharmacy would dispense mainly solutions for oral dosage.

Liquids for oral dosage are normally dispensed in plastic dispensing bottles which have markings on the side for milliliters, drams, ounces, or all three (for a review of dispensing units, see Chapter 11). The markings on a dispensing bottle are not accurate for measurement. They are a guide for the patient to determine approximately how much is left in the bottle. Never measure a solution or suspension by these markings. Solutions and suspensions must be measured at room temperature, using accurate devices (see Chapter 13).

Bulk Compounding and Bulk Manufacturing

Preparing a solution, ointment, or powder from a written procedure is called **bulk compounding**. Preparing a large volume (for example, solutions such as saline for irrigation) is called **bulk manufacturing**. Both must be prepared by the technician according to a standardized, written procedure in order to be legal. The procedure may involve combining the components by weight (see Chapter 21) or by percentages (see Chapter 12).

Preparing Sterile Solutions Using Aseptic Technique

If a sterile solution is being prepared, such as that for injection or use in surgical irrigation, the technician must practice **aseptic technique** (see Chapter 16). Since drugs which go directly into the blood or internal tissues do not go through the digestive system or lymph system, where bacteria will be destroyed, these preparations must be free of viruses, yeast, and bacteria. The human body is literally crawling with organisms which benefit the body by digesting food, flakes of old skin, and the like. Should these organisms get into the blood, however, they can cause a serious problem. The air that we breathe and the dirt under our feet (and fingernails) is also home to a huge number of bacteria, molds, and fungus, as well as parasites. We are filthy, from a bacterial point of view, and showering and scrubbing the skin will not remove these organisms. When we prepare an oral dosage, these organisms are not a problem, as long as we are clean. The acid in the stomach and the cells of the lymph system will take care of most organisms present in an oral medication. This is not true of a medication that bypasses the digestive system and enters directly into the blood. The high level of sugars and protein in the blood makes it an ideal breeding ground for microorganisms, and, because the immune system cannot keep up with the rate of their growth, the organisms can quickly cause **sepsis** ("blood poisoning") and death to the patient. Thus, when preparing a solution for parenteral use, extra care must be used. The following should be considered when preparing a solution for injection or admixture:

- All procedures should be performed inside of a sterile "laminar flow" hood with clean, disinfected hands, and the hair tied back. The sterile hood is a piece of equipment that surrounds the workspace and forms a barrier between the user/surroundings and the workspace. It electronically draws filtered room air across the front of the workspace from one side of the hood to the other ("horizontal flow") or pushes it forward from the back of the hood across the workspace and up to the top of the hood in a circle, creating a barrier from the workspace to the ceiling of the hood ("vertical flow") to keep organisms in the air away from the workspace. Air currents can still force organisms into the hood, however, so it should be kept away from traffic.

- The manufacturer's container, especially the site where the drug is to be withdrawn (or injected, as in the case of an admixture), must be disinfected with alcohol.

- Both the syringe and needle must be kept sterile. When inside the sterile packaging, the syringe and needle are guaranteed by the manufacturer to be sterile. When the packaging of the syringe is opened, it should be opened from the end that will attach to the needle, and care should be taken not to touch either the syringe or needle. The protective cap should be left on the needle at all times, unless the needle is being used to withdraw or inject the drug. Note that wearing latex gloves when working in the hood does not guarantee sterility, as they have been exposed to an unsterile environment.

- The top of the vial or manufacturer's container, where the needle is to be placed, should be disinfected with alcohol immediately before withdrawal.

- The needle should be placed at an angle of 45° with the top of the container, before insertion, as the end of the needle is "beveled" (cut and polished) to that angle. This helps to avoid "coring," getting the rubber from the septum (the "stopper") into the injection.

- When the medication is withdrawn, care must be taken not to touch the plunger on the syringe with your fingers as it is pulled out of the barrel. The plunger is going to go back into the barrel when the drug is ejected, and any organisms which are on it could get into the patient.

- After filling the syringe, the protective cap should be placed back over the needle before removal from the hood.

- Should the needle come in contact with the workspace or the side of the hood at any time, the entire assembly should be discarded.

Working With Hazardous Drugs

Additional measures must be taken if the drug is hazardous. Many injectable drugs, such as cancer chemotherapeutics and steroid drugs, can be harmful to the person handling them. So, in addition to keeping the drug sterile, as described above, the technician must wear protective clothing. This includes clothing that covers the body: no shorts, short-sleeved shirts, or skirts should be worn. In addition, a long protective coat (lab coat) should be worn to protect the clothing and person, and safety glasses or goggles should be worn to protect the eyes. Safety glasses should have splash guards on the sides, because when a drug is diluted within a vial, the pressure within the vial may build up, causing the drug to splash out if the vial is opened.

These coverings are for the protection of the technician, not the drug: they do not help to keep the drug sterile. If the drug is hazardous, the technician should also wear additional disposable body coverings such as a hat, mask, gloves, and shoe covers. This not only helps to prevent the drug from touching the skin but helps prevent contaminating the other parts of the pharmacy with the drug, as the coverings can be removed at the door of the IV room and discarded. When working with a sterile drug, particularly one that is hazardous, care should be taken to keep hands at least six inches inside of the hood, away from other parts of the body (see Chapter 23). Whether the drug is hazardous or not, touching the face or rubbing the eye is a source of contamination. This becomes even worse with a hazardous drug, as any contact with the face, particularly the mucous membranes of the eye and mouth, can introduce concentrated drug into the body in doses much larger than the patient would ever get. This can be extremely harmful. Similar precautions should be taken if the technician is allergic to the drug being prepared. Protective clothing, goggles, gloves, and mask should be worn when handling the medication.

Intravenous Admixtures and Injections

Various sites which may be used for drug injection, and each type of injection must be prepared in a different way (see Chapters 17 and 18). Intravenous injections may be high volume, as they go directly into the blood. Intramuscular injections have a limited volume, as there is not much room within the muscle for the drug to go. They also require a larger needle, as the muscle is tough and hard to inject. Intramuscular injections are designed to be released slowly from the muscle into the blood, whereas intravenous injections go directly into the blood. Subcutaneous injections are also designed for slow release of drug into the system and, since the space under the skin is also limited, have a relatively small volume. The very large volume injectables are the intravenous drips (IV drips). These are large plastic bags or glass bottles of solution, which may be used alone (for a dehydrated patient, for example) or with an **admixture**.

An IV admixture is a drug which is added to a large volume parenteral so that the drug is released slowly into the blood and is less of a shock to the body than a large "all-at-once" dose (a **bolus**). Admixtures are done in two ways. The drug to be administered may be in a separate, very small, IV bag which is designed to infuse slowly into the tubing with the IV drip. This is called a **piggyback IV**. Otherwise, the drug may be drawn up in the pharmacy (see Chapter 19) and injected into the IV bag or bottle, mixed by hand, and labeled appropriately, with the name of the solution, the name of the drug, the amount of drug added, and appropriate patient designation. When a sterile product, such as an IV bag or admixture, is labeled, the label should be placed toward the top of the container. This is so that any contamination present in the solution, which will tend to sink to the bottom of the container, can easily be seen. The contaminated product can then be discarded before it enters the patient. Labels on a syringe should be as narrow as possible and should be placed at the top of the syringe, crosswise, so as not to cover the markings on the syringe.

Auxiliary Labels

Once an outpatient prescription has been filled and labeled (since the medication will be dosed directly by the patient), it is helpful to place reminders on the prescription bottle as to how to use the medication and any activities that should be avoided while using it. These are called **auxiliary labels** and contain pictoral messages such as a sleepy eye ("May Cause Drowsiness") or a piece of bread ("Take with Food"). This reminds the patient of the best way to use the drug for maximum effect, and things to avoid which may be hazardous, such as drinking alcoholic beverages (which may chemically or physically react with the drug) or operating machinery. Once the drug has been dispensed and received by the patient, it now should be entered into the patient profile (Chapter 3).

Questions for Review

1. A prescription for Flexeril includes the instructions "i tab qd hs." What auxiliary label might be chosen to be affixed to the dispensing container?
   1. Take with food
   2. Drink with plenty of water
   3. May cause drowsiness
   4. For the eye

2. A drug suspension was removed from the refrigerator and a dose immediately measured out for the patient. The patient might receive:
   1. a lower dose of medication than prescribed.
   2. a higher dose of medication than prescribed
   3. the correct dose.
   4. drugs are not stored in the refrigerator.

3. An order is received for phenobarbital 50 mg po. The pharmacy has 100 mg tablets in stock. The order can only be filled if:
    1. the tablets are broken in half.
    2. the tablets are scored.
    3. the tablets are scored in half.
    4. the order cannot be filled, as the drug strengths do not match.

4. The dosage strength of the medication dispensed may not appear on the label if:
    1. the strength is below 10 mg.
    2. the drug is a combination drug.
    3. the drug only comes in one strength.
    4. both 2 and 3 are correct.

5. Which of the following are involved in the practice of aseptic technique?
    1. Clean hands
    2. Use of a laminar flow hood
    3. Alcohol disinfection
    4. All of the above

6. Aseptic technique is used for parenteral injections only, because:
    1. sterility is more important in drugs which enter directly into the body.
    2. any of the thousands of bacteria and fungus around us could cause serious infections if allowed into the bloodstream.
    3. bacteria and other organisms multiply rapidly once in the bloodstream and could cause death to the patient, and these organisms are destroyed by the digestive system.
    4. all of the above are true.
    5. none of the above—aseptic technique is important in all types of drug doses.

Solutions to Questions for Review

1. The instructions are to take one tablet at bedtime. This implies that the drug may make the patient drowsy. The correct answer is **3**.

2. Withdrawing and measuring a drug solution while it is cold may cause error, because when the drug is warmed to room temperature, it will expand. Thus the patient may be given a larger dose than prescribed, because the solution contracted at cold temperature and gave a deceptively low volume, which was actually greater when measured at the proper temperature. *It should be noted*, however, that some suspensions must be kept cold at all times, so some error is expected and factored into the dosage prescribed. The correct answer is **2**.

3. If the tablet is scored so that an accurate measurement of a partial tablet can be made, the prescription may be filled. Since one half of a tablet is needed, the tablets would have to be scored in half. The correct answer is **3**.

4. If the drug only comes in one strength, the strength does not need to be specified on either the prescription or the label. The same applies for combination drugs, which are drugs sold in combination with other drugs (e.g., Tylenol #3, trimethoprim, and sulfisoxazole, etc.). The correct answer is **4**.

5. Since aseptic means the cleanest possible, all of these practices would be used. The best answer is **4**.

6. While dispensing of any drug should be the cleanest possible, aseptic technique is used only for injectable drugs. **(1)** Sterility is extremely important for drugs injected into the body, because **(3)** organisms multiply in the bloodstream, causing sepsis (they are destroyed by the digestive system, if the drugs are taken orally), and these organisms come from **(2)** the surroundings. The correct answer is **4**.

Chapter 5

Proper Storage and Delivery of Drug Products

Quick Study

(See text for full explanation.)

I. **Drug *stability* and *potency***
   A. *Effects of humidity and air*
   B. *Importance of proper packaging* and packaging materials
   C. *Relationship of dosage form* to stability
   D. *The effects of temperature and light* on drug formulations
   E. Use of the manufacturer's label

II. **Handling the drug to be dispensed**
   A. *Calculation of drug concentration* from the manufacturer's label
   B. *Importance of cleanliness* in handling the drug
   - Drug allergies and sensitivities
   - Bacterial contamination

III. **Unit Dosing**
   A. Preparation of unit doses
   B. Use and care of *floor stock*: role of the technician and pharmacy
   - Inspection for cleanliness
   - Record keeping
   - Drug transfer and legal issues

Storage Conditions

Part of delivering an effective drug is related to the way the drug is stored in the warehouse and on the pharmacy shelf. Remember that drugs are chemicals; some are sensitive to light, others to heat, humidity, or oxygen in the air. Some drugs actually chemically react with their packaging; for example, nitroglycerine will react with plastic. A similar drug, sodium nitroprusside, will not only react with plastic but must be immediately protected from light (usually by covering the bottle with foil) once it has been reconstituted.

The form of the drug makes a difference as well. The stability of a drug (how well it retains its potency and form) is affected, as mentioned above, by things like water and air. Thus, a drug that is packaged dry on the shelf may retain potency longer than if water is added. The presence of water accelerates the breakdown of the drug and severely shortens the shelf life (although the rate of breakdown is slowed down by refrigeration; see below). A drug tablet is a pressed powder form which carries most of the drug inside of the tablet, protected from air and moisture. Thus, the tablet form may retain potency longer than a loose powdered form of the same drug, simply because less of the drug is exposed. Various storage conditions may help to protect the drug from breakdown. These include:

- **Opaque glass or plastic packaging**. Since the energy from light rays tends to speed up the breakdown (degradation) of most drug products, drugs are routinely packaged and dispensed in opaque bottles, or bottles made of brown plastic or glass. Even with the protective packaging, these drugs should be kept out of direct sunlight, and care must be taken to be sure that the container lid forms a tight seal against humidity and oxygen from the air, which can also destroy the drug.

- **Refrigeration**. Colder temperatures tend to slow down any chemical reaction, so as a rule, if drugs are refrigerated they may retain their potency longer (some drugs precipitate out in the cold, or may separate, so refrigeration might not be the best thing for all drugs; the manufacturer's label should be consulted). Additionally, sterile products are usually refrigerated, as colder temperatures will slow the growth of any contaminating organisms. Even a solution that is not meant for parenteral use may benefit from refrigeration, as keeping the solution cold may reduce the chance of breeding mold and fungi in the solution.

- **Dehydration**. Drugs in solution tend to break down faster than those in powder form. Some drugs are received in powder form for this reason (a longer shelf life) and are hydrated just before use. If a quantity of the drug must be stored in solution form (hydrated), its shelf life is limited, and much of the drug may have to be discarded before it can be sold. The shelf life of the hydrated drug may be extended by refrigeration, as refrigeration may slow the breakdown process (see above).

Determination of the Proper Storage Conditions for a Drug

The manufacturer's label on the stock bottle should be consulted to determine the proper storage conditions for a drug. The manufacturer's label, in addition to allowing us to accurately calculate the amount of drug dispensed per dose (Chapter 4), gives other information as well that is necessary for the proper handling of the drug (Figure 4–1).

The label contains information about the temperature at which the drug should be stored, and also states any storage conditions which should be avoided, such as heat, cold, light, or humidity. For example, if the label states "protect from light," the drug is light sensitive and should be stored appropriately. If it states "keep container tightly closed," the drug is sensitive to humidity or to the oxygen in the air. Normally this statement refers to exposure of the drug to humidity—many drugs will absorb water out of the air which decreases their potency. If there are no storage instructions, the drug should be stored at room temperature, away from bright light and heat.

The label may specify a specific temperature or range at which the drug should be stored. The technician must be familiar with what these temperatures mean, in terms of where, in the pharmacy, the drug should be stored. If the label refers to a temperature of

- 0°-5°C, the drug should be refrigerated.
- below 0°C, it refers to storage in the freezer. Usually, this is a warning (as to how the drug should not be stored), as most drugs are sensitive to extreme cold.
- 25°C or 75°F, refers to normal room temperature. The drug may be stored on the pharmacy shelf.

Label warnings might include the following:

- 30°C or 85°F (a "warm" room). Drugs will lose potency when exposed to heat.
- above 35°C or 95°F ("extreme heat"). This is too high a temperature for drug products.

Some drugs react chemically with plastic so will carry a warning to use only glass bottles. The label also provides information for proper handling (e.g., "shake well before using"). The dosage form is clearly stated on the label in Figure 4–1 as a suspension. (What does that mean in terms of handling the drug and drawing up the dose? Review Chapter 3.) The label also states the amount (volume) of suspension in the bottle. This is useful in two ways: first, it tells us how many doses we can draw out of the bottle. Second, and very important, if the concentration of the drug suspension or solution is not given on the bottle, it can be calculated by dividing the total amount of drug in the bottle by the total volume of drug solution in the bottle. Then, the proper amount for dispensing can be calculated.

Importance of Cleanliness and Sanitation During Storage

In addition to following the manufacturer's instructions when handling a drug, you must take care to keep the drug clean and sanitary. Dust on the bottle or shelves can contain molds, fungi, or bacteria that can contaminate the drug. Also, when a tablet counter or other measuring device is used, it is important to clean the device before and after each use to avoid **cross-contamination** of drugs. When more than one drug is handled at once, some residual drug may remain on the measuring device and will contaminate the second drug with another medication that may be harmful to the patient (even a trace of drug remaining on a counting tray could cause a severe allergic reaction, should the patient happen to be allergic to that drug), or, at the very least, that may react with or inactivate the drug.

Preparation of Unit Doses

A **unit dose** is part of a dosing system that is used in an institutional pharmacy. Simply stated, it is enough drug to last for a whole day. In an institution, it is more efficient to dispense an entire day's worth of medication at one time, to be administered by the floor staff, rather than order each individual dose from the pharmacy. This dose is calculated, dispensed, and, usually, delivered to the patient care area by the technician once a day. Unit doses are stored in a medication cart and are filed under patient name or hospital identification number (see Chapter 1).

A unit dose is calculated from the pharmacy order or MAR. The amount of medication per dose is multiplied by the number of doses per day (a twenty-four hour period). For example, if an order is for cimetidine 300 mg TID ac, the calculation would be:

$$1 \text{ tablet} \times 3 \text{ doses} = 3 \text{ tablets per day.}$$

This amount would be packaged appropriately and labeled with the patient's name, location, and hospital number as well as the drug name, strength, and form, if appropriate. Tablets may be packaged in blister packs ("bingo cards") or in another form that keeps the drug sanitary. Injectable medication may be sent in a prefilled syringe, vial, or dosette.

Exceptions to Unit Dosing

Exceptions to unit dosing include those medications that cannot be accurately measured for a unit dose, such as creams and ointments, and liquids for oral medication. These medications are sent to the patient floor in bulk, in a tube, jar, or bottle, as appropriate. When the exchange of medications takes place each day (unused medications are picked up and new doses delivered), these bulk medications are transferred from the previous day's medications to the current medications. *With the unit dose system, the patient is charged only for the medication that is used*, not for drugs that are picked up and returned to the pharmacy or for bulk medications that are not used.

Use of Pharmacy Inventory as Floor Stock

To further decrease the workload of the pharmacy and increase the availability of medication to the patient floors, the pharmacy may send drugs to patient floors to use as **floor stock**. In this case, the nurses station or emergency room would be responsible for keeping a supply of drugs and drug products that are normally needed within the unit itself. Drugs would then be used, inventoried, and ordered in large quantities from the pharmacy, by the personnel working in the unit. The pharmacy staff, however, is responsible for ensuring that the drugs are properly stored and dispensed. Periodic checks must be made to ensure the following:

- All drugs are being stored at the proper temperature. This may include measuring of the temperature of storage areas, such as refrigerators, as well as ensuring that drugs are stored appropriately, and in a sanitary manner, according to the manufacturer's label. This may also include checking to see if drugs that are to be refrigerated are being left on the counter when not in use. If this happens, the drug potency would be reduced and bacterial contamination may occur.
- Drugs are being dispensed properly, under sanitary conditions. Sloppy handling may lead to caps being left off of the stock bottles, exposing the drug to air, light, and humidity, which would lower the drug potency. In addition, this would expose the drug to dust and microorganisms in the air, such as bacteria, fungi, and viruses, causing contamination of the drug.

- The general environment of the dispensing area is clean and sanitary. No dirt, clutter, used syringes or needles, or contaminated materials should be present in the dispensing area (e.g., urine or blood specimens, or other laboratory specimens), nor should any food or drink be present.

- Proper records are being kept of drug utilization. Inventory of current stock, drugs dispensed to patients, and drugs ordered and received from the pharmacy must match. This is especially important with controlled substances, particularly Schedule II drugs. Any discrepancies must be reported immediately to the pharmacist and supervising professional.

Documenting Drug Transfer from the Pharmacy to Floor Stock Areas

Accurate records must be kept of the transfer of drugs from the control of the pharmacy to the control of the patient care area. When requested drugs are delivered to patient care areas, the technician must receive a signature of the person accepting the drugs and must provide a complete inventory of drugs delivered. If the delivery to the patient care area contains controlled substances, additional paperwork is required specifying the exact amount of drug to be transferred and including all information about the drug—the generic/proprietary name, manufacturer, lot number and expiration date of the drug, drug dosage, and dosage form. The signature of the head nurse or supervising medical professional is required for delivery of any controlled substance (Schedule drug) to be used as floor stock outside of the main pharmacy. A signature by any other person is not acceptable. The receipt of the drug(s) by the patient care area is acknowledged by this signature, and responsibility for the disposition and records involving the drugs is transferred at this time.

Questions for Review

1. The best way to determine the storage conditions for a particular drug is to:
   1. ask the pharmacist.
   2. refer to the *United States Pharmacopoeia*.
   3. try different ways of storage.
   4. refer to the manufacturer's label.

2. The stability of a drug refers to:
   1. whether it reacts with plastic.
   2. how long it can be stored on the pharmacy shelf.
   3. how long it remains potent.
   4. how it should be stored.

3. A reconstituted drug in suspension:
   1. is more stable than a dry powder.
   2. is normally stored on the pharmacy shelf.
   3. will remain potent longer if it is refrigerated.
   4. will slowly break down over time

4. You have a bottle of drug in solution. The label does not state the concentration of the drug in the solution, but the amount of drug and the volume of liquid in the container both appear on the label. To dispense 30 mg of this drug, you can:
   1. obtain further information from the pharmacopoeia.
   2. estimate the amount of drug to be dispensed by the volume needed for injection.
   3. calculate the concentration from the information given on the label.
   4. the order cannot be filled.

5. Contamination of dispensed drugs may occur from:
   1. dust clinging to the bottle and cap falling into the medication.
   2. residual drug clinging to the measuring device, which has not been properly cleaned.
   3. unfiltered room air.
   4. not using a laminar flow hood when dispensing the medication.
   5. both 1 and 2 could be correct.

6. Drugs in inventory that are "slow movers" should be:
   1. ordered less frequently.
   2. removed from inventory.
   3. reduced in price.
   4. put in a special area.

7. You receive an order for cefaclor 250 mg ii bid. The drug is available in 250 mg capsules. A unit dose for this patient would be:
   1. two capsules.
   2. three capsules.
   3. four capsules.
   4. this drug could not be dispensed as a unit dose.

8. Which of the following would not be dispensed as a unit dose?
   1. Cimetidine tablets
   2. Verapamil capsules
   3. Phenergan syrup
   4. Perchlorphenazine suppositories

9. A drug label says to store the drug between 15 and 25 degrees centigrade. The drug should be stored:
   1. in a warm room.
   2. on the pharmacy shelf.
   3. in the refrigerator.
   4. in a cool room.
   5. in the freezer.

Solutions to Questions for Review

1. Each drug has a particular storage "preference," the conditions under which it will retain the most potency. As a rule, medications will stay potent longer if shielded from light, heat, and humidity. To determine the best conditions for a particular drug and the form which it is in, it is best to **(4)** consult the manufacturer's label.

2. The stability of a drug refers to how fast it will break down. Once it begins to break down, it loses potency and will not work as well at prescribed doses. The correct answer is **3**.

3. A reconstituted drug in suspension is mixed with water. Hydrating the drug causes the drug to be less stable and lose potency at a faster rate. The main thing which will slow this process is **(3)** refrigeration. Since **2** refers to storage at 25°C, and refrigerated temperature is 5°C, storage on the pharmacy shelf would not be advisable. Since drugs in suspension tend to break down more quickly, **4** would also be incorrect. The correct answer is **3**.

4. If the strength of a drug solution or suspension is not given on the label, it can be easily calculated. Simply divide the volume by the total amount of drug. The correct answer is **3**.

5. Contamination of drugs may arise from microorganisms in the air and room dust, as well as dirt and other sources. The amount of contamination from room air is not a problem for drugs that are not meant for parenteral use, so **3** would be incorrect. However, improper cleaning of measuring devices can lead to contamination of a dispensed drug, not with microorganisms but with another drug. The correct answer is **5**

6. Slow-moving drugs are still prescribed and thus should be kept in inventory. However, to maintain an efficient system of inventory, they should be ordered in smaller quantities and less frequently. The correct answer is **1**.

7. A unit dose is drug sufficient for twenty-four hours. Since the order is for two capsules taken twice a day, the unit dose is 2×2 or four capsules. The correct answer is **3**.

8. If a drug cannot accurately be measured out and administered as a unit dose, it is packaged as a "non-unit dose" medication. Since all of the medications are "countable," with the exception of the phenergan syrup, the correct answer is **3**.

9. 25°C is room temperature, and 5°C is refrigeration. Therefore, 15°C would be a cool room. The correct answer is **4**.

Chapter 6

Receiving Monetary Compensation for Goods and Services

Quick Study

(See text for full explanation)

I. **Payment for pharmacy services**
   A. *Self pay*
   B. *Third party payer*
   - Direct payment to pharmacy ("co-pay")
   - "Out-of-pocket" (reimbursement to patient)
   C. Benefits and limitations

II. **Profit and markup: calculation of selling price and net profit**

Methods of Payment for Pharmacy Services

There are basically two ways in which the pharmacy can receive payment for services. One is **self-pay**, in which the patient pays the pharmacy directly. The second is payment by a **third-party payer**. The third-party payer can be used in two ways: (1) the patient can pay the pharmacy and be reimbursed (**out-of-pocket**), in which case the pharmacist must fill out an insurance affidavit stating the drugs received, price, and other information required by the insurance company, or (2) the patient can pay a small amount (**co-payment** or **co-pay**) and the pharmacy bills the insurance for the balance of the price.

Third-Party Payers—Benefits and Exclusions

The technician needs to be familiar with the billing of third party payers. These payers may include:

- traditional insurance companies such as those received under an employee benefit package
- govenment plans such as Medicare and Medicaid
- private insurance companies.

Each care plan has specific benefits and may or may not include payments for medications. Those plans which cover prescription medications may limit coverage in various ways, such as excluding outpatient prescriptions, limitation of outpatient coverage to oral dosage forms, exclusion of proprietary drugs, or limitations on quantity. The technician must be familiar with the various plans and what they cover. Normally, when the insurance is verified at the time that the prescription is received, information displayed by the pharmacy computer program includes the coverage. If the plan allows only generic drugs to be dispensed and the patient or prescriber requests a brand-name (proprietary) label, the patient would have to make up the difference in price. Exceptions to policy may be made by the insurance company, under certain circumstances (e.g., the condition is life threatening or there is no generic brand available).

Once insurance coverage or method of payment has been established, the forms to be submitted to the insurance company must be identified and completed and the price of the medication calculated. The selling price of a medication begins with the cost of the medication to the pharmacy (**cost price**). This is then placed in a formula that computes the price, based on markup (see Chapter 9). All medications dispensed by prescription will also include a **dispensing fee**. This may either be a percentage of the price or a flat fee added to the cost of the prescription.

Institutional Pharmacy Billing

In an institutional pharmacy setting, the technician does not fill out insurance forms or bill insurance directly. Instead, charges are billed to the patient's account, using the patient profile and medication administration record (MAR) as a record of medications and supplies dispensed. Normally, charges are billed to the patient's account at the time the medication is dispensed, which simplifies the billing process and improves billing accuracy. Insurance coverage verification and billing, in a hospital setting, are normally done by a separate billing or accounting department within the institution.

Profit and Markup

The **markup** of a drug is normally expressed as a percentage of the cost. For example, a markup of 100% would mean that the increase in price would be equal to the cost. (Since 100% is the same as multiplying a number by one, the markup is the same as the cost.) The markup of a drug is the same as the profit that is made on the drug (which is usually expressed in dollars and cents). If a drug costs $2 and we mark it up 100%, the markup is then 1 × $2, or $2 profit. For a discussion of the calculation of selling price, see Chapter 9.

Questions for Review

1. The two types of third-party pay plans are:
   1. co-pay and self pay.
   2. co-pay and out-of-pocket.
   3. reimbursement and self-pay.
   4. bill-to and reimbursement.

2. The insurance affidavit:
   1. is a sworn contract to pay charges.
   2. is a document that is filled out so that the pharmacy gets paid.
   3. must be completed by the pharmacist.
   4. is completed by the patient and sent to the insurance company.

3. An example of a third-party payer would not be:
   1. Medicare.
   2. Medicaid.
   3. a man ordered to pay medical expenses as a result of a lawsuit.
   4. a major insurance company.

4. The selling price of a medication is based on the:
   1. patient's income.
   2. amount the insurance will pay.
   3. cost price to the pharmacy.
   4. dispensing fee.

Solutions to Questions for Review

1. When a portion is paid by the patient, it is co-pay. When the patient is reimbursed, it is called out-of-pocket, as the patient must pay first before being reimbursed. The correct answer is **2**.

2. The insurance affidavit is a form filled out by the pharmacist, which is sent to the insurance company by the patient who is then reimbursed. The pharmacy is paid when the prescription is filled. The correct answer is **3**.

3. A third-party payer is an organization which is in the business of insurance. This would include union plans, employee insurance, health benefits, Medicare, and Medicaid. The correct answer is **3**.

4. To compute the selling price of a medication, we must first take the pharmacy's cost and mark up the price by a percentage of that cost. The correct answer is **3**.

SECTION II

Inventory Control

Chapter 7   Stocking the Pharmacy

Chapter 8   Maintenance of Drug Products

Chapter 9   Commercial Calculations

Stocking the Pharmacy

Quick Study

(See text for full explanation.)

I. **Choosing the drug formulary**

    A. Drug *cost*, *efficacy*, and the *frequency of prescription* (drug demand)

    B. *Uses, adverse effects*, and *storage requirements* of a drug

II. **Ordering and receipt of drugs and devices**

    A. Use of the *purchase order* and *"want book"*

    B. Information to be specified when ordering drugs and devices

- The *drug* or *device name* (generic or proprietary)
- *Strength* and *dosage form* of the drug (or *size*, if ordering a device)
- *Quantity per package* of drug dosage forms and packaging type
- *Quantity ordered* of bottles, packages, or devices

III. **Ordering of controlled substances: Schedules II-IV**

The Drug Formulary

The list of drugs that reflects what the pharmacy routinely stocks is called a **formulary**. There are literally hundreds of individual drugs available for dispensing by the pharmacy, and the pharmacy cannot possibly stock all available drugs. The pharmacy must choose which drugs to stock, based on cost, efficacy (how well the drug works), and demand. The national formulary is a listing of all drugs marketed in the United States. The letters NF after a drug name indicate that the drug is included in the national formulary.

The drug formulary within an institution is derived by a joint effort of the pharmacist and the institution. In a hospital pharmacy, an organization within the hospital called the *Pharmacy and Therapeutics Committee* decides which drugs to stock in the pharmacy. This committee is made up of the pharmacist and representatives of the various health care fields: a physician, nurse, and dietitian. This is necessary to present all views on the ease of use and efficacy of a drug, in order to choose the best drugs to stock. For example, one drug may be just as efficacious as another but very difficult to administer or not well tolerated by the patient. The pharmacist does not have contact with the patients to actually administer the medication, so other professionals are needed to accurately assess the drugs.

The formulary is a very selective list of drugs. These drugs have been selected because they have been determined to be *the best drugs at the lowest cost*. More than one proprietary (brand) name of a drug is available for most drugs, and many different generic brands are available as well. However, only one brand name and one generic per drug are normally stocked in a pharmacy, as stocking more than one brand of the same drug (called **drug duplication**) takes up valuable shelf space and resources. Two brands may be stocked, if there is sufficient justification for carrying both.

We choose which of the available drugs to stock in the pharmacy according to cost and efficacy, but the demand for the drug is also important. If only a few prescriptions are written for a particular drug, there is little sense in stocking it, as it costs the pharmacy money to maintain the drug on the pharmacy shelf (as discussed below). Other factors involved in the selection of drugs are their uses, side effects, and storage requirements. The storage requirements determine how much it will cost the pharmacy to keep the drug stocked ("carrying costs"). For example, if a particular drug is stored on the pharmacy shelf and another must be refrigerated, the one stored on the shelf would cost less to maintain.

The drug formulary is under constant revision. New drugs and dosage forms are constantly being produced, and as more information is gathered about older drugs, some may be removed from the market for unforseen problems.

Ordering and Receipt of Drug Products and Devices

Regular (nonschedule) drugs, devices (e.g., glucometers or other necessary measuring devices), and supplies (syringes, oral dosage devices, needles, and bandages) may be ordered electronically, by fax, modem, or computer. The order is normally made on a form called a **purchase order**. The decision to order a drug or item depends on how well it sells in the pharmacy. When the amount of a popular drug that sells quickly falls to 1,000 tablets on the shelf, for example, the drug may be reordered. The amount of a less popular drug may have to be substantially lower before reordering, perhaps 100 tablets remaining. Many pharmacies have a list of drugs and devices that routinely need to be ordered, called the "Want Book"—when the supply of a drug or device falls to the "reorder" point, it is entered into this list for reorder (ordering may be done routinely on a certain day of the week, for example, not whenever the stock of a drug falls low).

Ordering Regular Drugs and Devices

To order regular drugs, the **purchase order** is used. This form contains the information discussed above, as well as other information such as the vendor (the company selling the drug), price, shipping information, and date of order. The purchase order is usually assigned a number (the **purchase order number**) for tracking the shipment. The order is transmitted to the company, which generates a bill, or **invoice**, which tells the pharmacy how much to pay. The information on the invoice should be carefully checked against the purchase order, to be sure that the drug ordered and the drug that the pharmacy is being billed for are exactly the same in name, strength, and quantity.

Information to be specified when ordering includes the following:

- The drug or device name and manufacturer. For a drug product, the generic or brand (trade) name must be specified.
- The strength and dosage form of the drug (or size, if ordering a device).
- The quantity of drug dosage forms per package (e.g., bottle of 100, package of two).
- The type of packaging.
- The number of bottles, packages, or devices being ordered.

Drugs and supplies should be ordered in an organized and timely manner. Thus, the usual time for delivery should be taken into account when ordering. If the supplier takes three weeks to send a shipment of drugs to the pharmacy, the supply at the time of order cannot be so low that the pharmacy will run out before the shipment is received.

In case of emergency, when drugs or supplies are needed quickly, the technician must know of other sources from which to obtain the materials. In a pharmacy chain, this may be another pharmacy within the chain. In a hospital situation, drugs or urgent supplies may be "borrowed" from another hospital and replaced when reordered.

Ordering Controlled Substances (Schedule Drugs)

The technician may order regular drugs and devices for sale but may not order controlled substances, specifically Schedule II drugs. This may only be done by the pharmacist and requires a special triplicate form for ordering, called a DEA 41 form, which must be obtained from the Drug Enforcement Agency (DEA). The forms for ordering may only be obtained by a licensed health professional, such as a pharmacist, physician, or dentist. These forms are regulated and numbered, and records are kept of the numbers and to whom they were given. This security measure is intended to help prevent unauthorized persons from ordering controlled substances.

Questions for Review

1. The listing of drugs that are stocked in the pharmacy is called a(n):
   1. inventory.
   2. formulary.
   3. want list.
   4. dispensing list.

2. For each drug, a pharmacy normally stocks:
   1. all of the best trade names.
   2. all of the best generic brands.
   3. trade names and generic brands that are prescribed most frequently.
   4. only one trade name and one generic per drug.

3. Stocking more than one brand of the same drug is called:
   1. overstock.
   2. therapeutic duplication.
   3. drug duplication.
   4. residual stocking.

4. When the stock of drugs or supplies is low, a notation to reorder is placed into the:
   1. reorder list.
   2. want book.
   3. computer for reorder.
   4. reordering is usually done immediately.

5. Ordering of morphine tablets:
   1. may be done by the technician.
   2. is done by computer.
   3. requires a special form.
   4. must be done within five days of running out.
   5. both 1 and 4.

6. Which of the following must appear on a purchase order for a drug?
   1. The name of the drug
   2. The strength of drug
   3. The type of packaging and units per package
   4. All of the above

Solutions to Questions for Review

1. The pharmacy and the therapeutics committee or institution choose which drugs to stock and includes them in the formulary. The correct answer is **2**.

2. The decision of which drugs to stock is done by choosing the one trade name and one generic that are determined to be the best. The correct answer is **4**.

3. If more than one of the same drug is stocked, it is called drug duplication. Therapeutic duplication is when the patient is prescribed more than one of the same drug (usually under different names). The correct answer is **3**.

4. Drugs for reorder are placed into a Want Book for reorder at a later time. The correct answer is **2**.

5. Controlled substances, particularly Schedule II drugs, must be ordered by the pharmacist, using a triplicate DEA 41 form. The correct answer is **3**.

6. A purchase order for a drug must contain as much specific information about the drug, strength, and type of packaging as possible. The correct answer is **4**.

Chapter 8

Maintenance of Drug Products

Quick Study

(See text for full explanation.)

I. **Placing a drug in inventory**

    A. Use of the *national drug code (NDC number)*

    B. Routine inventories of regular drugs and drugs classified under Schedules II–IV

II. **Drug expiration and shelf life**

    A. Routine check for *expiration date* and *date of removal* from inventory

    B. Dispensing of drugs in close proximity to expiry date

    C. Disposition of expired drugs

        • Discarding of drugs by the pharmacist

        • Return for manufacturer's credit

III. **Drug recalls**

    A. *Notification of patients and prescibers*

    B. *Recapture* of recalled drug products dispensed

IV. **Drug recapture**

    A. Disposition of recaptured drugs - institutional vs. retail pharmacies

    B. Proper disposal of contaminated drugs—role of the pharmacist

V. **Comparing procedures in retail and institutional settings**

Maintenance of Drug Products in Inventory

Once the drugs are received, they are placed in inventory. This means that the drug name, strength, and quantity must be entered into the computer system. Drugs are identified using a series of numbers printed on the stock bottle label, called a **national drug code (NDC) number**. This number identifies the drug, the specific dosage form, the strength, and the manufacturer. The amount of tablets (or number of milliliters, etc.) must be entered into the records, and the amount dispensed is normally deducted from inventory electronically. A physical inventory of the regular prescription drugs must be conducted every five years, and a complete inventory of controlled substances must be made every two years.

Importance of Proper Storage of Drug Products in Inventory

During the time that drugs remain in inventory, they must be stored properly, in a way which maintains the integrity of the drug. Drugs and drug products must be stored in a climate-controlled environment. Climate control includes low levels of light and humidity and proper temperature. During storage, drugs must be kept clean, sanitary, and up-to-date. This means that the drug containers should be free of dust and kept away from light and humidity. Drugs in inventory must also be checked at regular intervals for proximity to expiration dates. Those which are close to expiration should be removed from inventory.

Rotation of Stock

Once drugs have been properly stored, it is important when adding new inventory to place the newest product toward the back of the storage area so that the older drugs, which are closer to expiration, will be dispensed first. This is called rotation of stock, and helps to keep drugs from getting too close to their expiration dates before they are dispensed.

Storage of Controlled Drugs (Schedule Drugs)

It is also important to remember that, although regular drugs may be stored on the pharmacy shelf or in areas with free access, drugs under Schedules II to IV, particularly Schedule II drugs, must be stored in a locked cabinet or storage area. This is a security measure to prevent unlawful procurement of such drugs by unauthorized personnel. Since the pharmacist is legally responsible for any discrepancies in inventory when the records of the pharmacy are audited, the pharmacist usually retains the key.

Handling Expired Medications and Drug Recalls

Medications in inventory must be routinely checked for proximity to their expiration date. Once a product is within a few weeks of expiration (preferably within six months), it must be removed from the shelves.

Legally, a drug may be sold up to and on the date of expiration, but it is good practice to remove drugs from the pharmacy shelves prior to that date, as the patient may retain the drug for as much as a month or more before finishing the prescription, during which time the drug could pass its expiration date. Expired drugs may be discarded with proper documentation but are often returned to the manufacturer for credit. Disposal of drug products requires documentation for the DEA and is done by the pharmacist.

Occasionally, a drug product may be contaminated, produced improperly, or is deemed to have unexpected or detrimental side effects. In this case, the Food and Drug Administration (FDA) mandates a **recall** of the drug or a specific drug lot found to have a problem. Not only is the drug pulled from the shelves and returned to the manufacturer, with appropriate documentation, but dispensing records must also be examined to determine which patients have received that particular drug or particular lot of drug. These patients must be contacted and advised to return their prescriptions to the pharmacy for exchange. Returned drug products are then documented and returned to the manufacturer for credit. In addition to the patients receiving the drug, the prescribers must also be notified of the problem in order to halt prescription of the recalled drug.

Drug "Recapture"

In a retail pharmacy, drugs and devices may not be returned once they leave the control of the pharmacy. However, in an institutional setting, the pharmacy may receive returned drugs from unit dose medications which were not used. These medications, if unopened, may be replaced in inventory. Drugs which have been opened, such as drug vials from which medication has been removed for a patient, are discarded according to procedure. Disposal of drugs is the responsibility of the pharmacist, as the drugs are toxic and an environmental hazard if not disposed of properly.

Questions for Review

1. When a drug is recalled, which of the following should occur?
   1. The patients using the drug should be notified.
   2. The providers prescribing the drug should be notified.
   3. The drug supply with the appropriate lot number should be removed from inventory and returned to the supplier.
   4. All of the above.

2. Unused unit dose medications:
   1. are always discarded.
   2. are reused for the next patient.
   3. may be placed back into inventory if unopened, and the charges credited back to the patient.
   4. may be distributed to floor nursing staff for emergency use.

3. A drug is found on the shelf that expires in three months. This drug:
   1. is OK to sell.
   2. should be sent back to the manufacturer.
   3. should be marked and reevaluated in three months.
   4. should be removed from the pharmacy shelf.

4. A complete inventory of regular prescription drugs:
   1. should be done every two years.
   2. should be done weekly.
   3. must be done every five years.
   4. should be done before every inspection by the DEA.

5. Controlled substances must be:
   1. kept in a locked cabinet.
   2. documented carefully, with no mistakes or strikeovers.
   3. inventoried every two years.
   4. all of the above.

6. Drugs on the shelf are stored in opaque bottles and dispensed in amber dispensing bottles because:
   1. the drugs are sensitive to heat.
   2. the drugs are sensitive to humidity.
   3. the drugs are sensitive to light.
   4. it is easier to handle that way.

Solutions to Questions for Review

1. In the case of a drug recall, affected drugs are identified by lot number and removed from the shelves to be returned to the supplier. All persons involved with the drug must be notified, including the patient and prescriber. The correct answer is **4.**

2. Unit dose medications, if unopened (and thus not contaminated), may be returned to inventory. The correct answer is **3.**

3. Drugs should be removed from the pharmacy shelf within six months before expiration. The correct answer is **4.**

4. Regular prescription drugs must be inventoried every five years. The correct answer is **3.**

5. Controlled substances must be inventoried every two years. They must also be kept separate, in a locked cabinet, and carefully documented. The correct answer is **4.**

6. Opaque bottles are used to protect the drug from light. The correct answer is **3.**

Chapter 9

Commercial Calculations

Quick Study

(See text for full explanation.)

I. **Computation of the selling price of a drug or device**
   A. Cost of the drug or device to the pharmacy *"cost price"*
   B. *Markup:* the percentage of the cost price which is added to the cost price (*markup = profit*)
   C. **Cost + Markup = Selling Price**

II. **Computation of dispensing charges**
   A. By percentage
   B. Using a flat dispensing fee

III. **Computation of sale prices**
   A. Selling price reduction by percent
   B. Loss of profit from sale reduction

Cost and Markup

In the pharmacy, prescription and over-the-counter drugs are normally ordered in large amounts (by the case or gross), in order to get a lower price. The *price that the pharmacy pays for a drug* or supply item is called the **cost price**. The drug or item cannot then be sold at the same price that was paid for it—there would be no profit to the pharmacy, which, after all, is a business. So, a *percentage of the cost price* (the **markup**) is added. Thus, when the pharmacy sells the item it makes a *profit*.

Calculating the Selling Price

Let's say you went to the store and bought a pound of potatoes. What you paid would be the cost price. Then, you take these potatoes to your neighbor, and sell them for twice what you paid for them. The extra amount that you charge your neighbor over what you paid for them (which, in this case, would be the same as what you paid for them, since you are charging him double the price) would be the markup on the potatoes. In this case, the markup is 100% (one times the cost). The amount that you charge your neighbor would be the **selling price**. Let's try a problem

The pharmacy buys a case of cold remedy for $20 (this is the cost price). It marks the price up by 100% (this is the markup). Multiplying by 100% is the same as multiplying by one (see Chapter 12). So, the amount which we add to the cost price before selling the item is an extra $20. To get the price we sell the item for (selling price), we add the two together. The selling price is:

COST ($20) + MARKUP ($20) = SELLING PRICE ($40)

This is an important formula to remember. With slight variations, all of the commercial calculations use this formula. For example, we can make the problem we just did more complicated. Normally, we do not sell products from the pharmacy by the case. We sell them individually. So, let's take the same problem and compute the selling price of each individual bottle of cold remedy.

To calculate prices for individual items, we must know not only the price of the case but also how many items there are per case. If there are 20 bottles of cold remedy in a case, and the cost price to the pharmacy is $20, that means that each bottle costs $1 ($20 ÷ 20 bottles). The markup is the same: 100%, or $1. So, the selling price is $1 + $1 = $2 per bottle.

The same goes for prescription drugs. Say we buy a stock bottle of Tegretol, which contains 1,000 tablets. It costs $250. The cost per tablet is $250 ÷ 1,000 = 25¢ per tablet. The markup is determined by the cost to store, maintain, and dispense the drug. Let's make it 200%. So, the charge per tablet is then 25¢ (cost) + (2 × 25¢) (markup) = 75¢ per tablet.

Twenty tablets would then cost $15. However, the pharmacy usually adds an additional amount—a **dispensing fee**—to each prescription, regardless of the size of the prescription. This is usually a flat fee, but it may be a percentage of the total price. So, the price of the 20 tablets, with a $5 dispensing fee, would cost $20 instead of $15. With a 5 percent dispensing fee, the cost would be $15 + (0.05 × $15) = $15.75. A pharmacy dispensing small prescriptions, as a rule, would benefit more from a flat fee system, and one selling mainly large quantities would benefit more from the percentage system. The type of dispensing fee is chosen by the institution (i.e., hospital or chain pharmacy).

Problems for Practice

1. A pharmacy sells a tube of Ben-Gay for $6.90, with a 200% markup. What was the cost of the Ben-Gay to the pharmacy?

2. Referring to question 1, how much profit will the pharmacy make on a case of 50 if it sells the Ben-Gay for 50% off?

3. You have a vial of ampicillin sodium for injection, containing 5 g of drug. You dilute it to 500 mg/ml. The cost of the vial is $15, and markup is 200%.
   a.   How much does the entire vial sell for?
   b.   How much profit will be made on the one vial?

4. You get an order for ampicillin sodium, 1 g IV bid. Disregarding dispensing fees, how much would the patient be billed for one dose? For a unit dose? (Hint: use the information from question 3.)

5. How much profit would the pharmacy make on a single dose for this patient?

6. You have a 10% solution of calcium gluconate, priced at $2 per 10 ml. There is a 200% markup on the drug product. Your order is for 1 g of calcium gluconate in a saline drip.
   a.   What would the patient be charged for the drug?
   b.   How much profit would the pharmacy make on this dose?

Solutions to Problems for Practice

1. Use the formula: COST + MARKUP = SELLING PRICE, cost = unknown, markup = 200%, or 2× cost, and selling price = $6.90. Fill in the equation:

$$\text{Cost} + 2\times \text{cost} = \$6.90$$

and solve for cost

$$\text{Cost} + 2\times \text{cost} = 3\times \text{cost} = \$6.90.$$

Divide both sides by 3 to get the cost

$$\frac{3\times \text{cost}}{3} = \frac{\$6.90}{3}$$

Cost is then $6.90 ÷ 3 or **$2.30 per tube.**

2. Remember: *profit* and *markup* are the same thing. If the original selling price is $6.90, half off of that (50% off) would be the new price, or $3.45 The cost price never changes—it is still $2.30. Therefore, the profit per tube is $3.45–2.30, or $1.15. There are 50 tubes, so total profit is 50 × $1.15 = **$57.50.**

3. a. Remember: a 200% markup means the same as two times the cost.

$$\text{COST of the vial} + \text{MARKUP} = \text{SELLING PRICE for the vial}$$
$$\$15 \;+\; 2 \;\times\; \$15 \;=\; \textbf{\$45 per vial.}$$

   b. The profit made on one vial = the markup = 2 × $15 = $30.

4. The vial contains 5 g of drug. The order is for 1 g, so 1 g/5 g, or 1/5 of the vial, will be dispensed for the patient. The vial sells for $45. So, 1/5 vial used × $45/vial = **$9/dose**. Since the patient receives the dose twice per day, the unit dose charge would be $9 × 2, or $18.

5. The patient is charged $9 per dose, and the drug has a 200% markup. Therefore, since COST + MARKUP = SELLING PRICE, 3 × the cost = $9. The cost = $9 ÷ 3, or $3, so the profit per dose is 2 × the cost (200%) = **$6.**

6. To figure the selling price (charged to the patient): A 10% solution is 10 g per 100 ml. A 1 g dose would be 1/10 of that 100 ml, or 10 ml. The solution is priced at $2 per 10 ml. Since 10 ml = the 1 g dose, the patient charge would be $2. To figure the profit made, we use the formula:

$$\text{COST} + \text{MARKUP} = \text{SELLING PRICE.}$$

Fill in the numbers:

$$\text{cost} + 2 \times \text{cost} = \$2,$$
$$\text{so } 3 \times \text{cost} = \text{selling price (\$2).}$$

The cost to the pharmacy is $2 ÷ 3, or 67¢. Since we are charging $2 per dose, the profit is $2–$0.67, or **$1.33.**

Pharmaceutical Calculations

Chapter 10 Fractions, Decimals, and Algebra Review

Chapter 11 Systems of Measurement

Chapter 12 Using Percentages and Ratios

Chapter 13 Measuring Equipment

Chapter 14 Conversion of Solid Dosage Forms

Chapter 15 Conversion of Liquid Dosage Forms

Chapter 16 Pediatric Doses

Chapter 17 Parenteral Dosages

Chapter 18 Intravenous Calculations

Chapter 19 Intravenous Admixtures

Chapter 20 Calculation of Dose per Time

Chapter 21 Bulk Compounding

Chapter 22 Math Test with Solutions

Chapter 10

Fractions, Decimals, and Algebra Review

Quick Study

(See text for full explanation.)

I. **Proper and improper fractions**

A. *Proper fraction*: the numerator is smaller than the denominator

B. *Improper fraction*: the numerator is greater than the denominator

II. **Addition and subtraction of fractions**: finding the common denominator and performing the calculation: $1/4 + 1/2 = 1/4 + 2/4 = 3/4$

$$1/2 - 1/4 = 2/4 - 1/4 = 1/4$$

III. **Multiplication of fractions**: multiplying numerators and multiplying denominators, then reducing the fraction, if necessary: $3/4 \times 1/2 = 3/8$

IV. **Division of fractions**

A. *Dividing the numerator* of one fraction by the numerator of another, then dividing the denominators in the same way: $3/4 \div 1/2 = (3 \div 1)/(4 \div 2) = 3/2 = 1\ 1/2$

B. Flipping over either fraction and multiplying: $3/4 \div 1/2 = 4/3 \times 1/2$ (or $3/4 \times 2/1$)

V. **Decimals**: fractions expressed in terms of tenths

A. $1/10 = 0.1$, $1/100 = 0.01$, $1/1000 = 0.001$

B. *Divide the numerator of a fraction by the denominator and express as a decimal*: $3/4 = 3 \div 4 = 0.75$. (Always place the zero in front of the decimal point, so that the number is not misinterpreted; .75 may look somewhat like a decimal, but the "point" could be a spot on the paper)

VI. **Working with decimals**: addition, subtraction (fixed decimal place), multiplication, and division

Dividing a Whole: Using Fractions

What is a fraction?

A fraction is nothing more than a part of a whole thing. Say we have a drug order for phenobarbital, 15 mg per dose. All we have in the pharmacy are 60 mg tablets and 100 mg tablets. We could send the patient to another pharmacy, but that's not good for either the pharmacy or the patient. So, we need to figure out how to make what we have in the pharmacy match what the doctor wants the patient to take. For that, we need fractions.

A fraction is arranged with a number on the top and on the bottom. The top number tells us how many of the total parts that we have. The bottom number tells us how many parts are in the whole thing. For example, if we have 1/2 tablet, we have one part of the total of two that make up the whole tablet. If we have 1/4 tablet, we have one of the four parts that make up a whole, and if we have a whole tablet, we have one part of a total of one part, or 1/1. If the top and bottom numbers are the same, four parts out of four (4/4) or three parts out of three (3/3), for example, we have the whole thing, so the fraction is equal to one. If you think of fractions as parts of a whole thing, pharmaceutical calculations will be much easier.

Writing Fractions

The correct way to write a fraction is with the top number smaller than the bottom (e.g., 1/2). If the top number is larger than the bottom number, it is called an **improper fraction** and the number is more than one. So (to be "proper") we should write this number as both a whole number and a fraction (1 3/4, for example). This is called a **mixed fraction**.

Adding Fractions

To add two fractions together, we must have a **common denominator** (the bottom parts of each fraction must be the same). Once the fractions have a common denominator, we can add the top parts together, reduce, and get the answer.

Example: 1/4 + 1/2

Step 1: The common denominator. We have two choices for the calculation of a common denominator: we can make the 2 in the "1/2" the same as the 4 in the "1/4," or do the opposite, and make the 4 into a 2.

Remember that whatever we do to the bottom number we also must do to the top number (if we do the same thing to both the top and bottom numbers, it's the same as multiplying the fraction by 1).

To be able to add the numbers, we must do one of these things. If we divide the 4 in the "1/4" by 2, we must divide the 1 also, and we would have a very strange number — 1/2 ÷ 2. So, we choose the other method: multiply the 2 in the "1/2" by 2, to make 4, and then multiply the 1 on the top, as well. This gives us 2/4, that is much better. Always pick the method which gives the easiest number to work with.

Step 2: Now that the bottom numbers are the same, we just add the top numbers: **1/4 + 2/4 = 3/4.**

Subtracting Fractions

This is done in the same way as addition, except that instead of adding the top numbers we subtract them.

Example: 2/3 – 1/2

Step 1: It is harder to get the bottom numbers the same this time, since neither of the numbers is divisible by the other. This time, the best way is to multiply the 3 by 2 and the 2 by 3 to get a common denominator: 2/3 × **2/2** = 4/6, and 1/2 x **3/3** = 3/6.

Now, we write the problem over again, and subtract the top numbers: 4/6 – 3/6 = 1/6. *It is important to get in the habit of re-writing the problem each time you work with the parts of it.* Memory is faulty, and, this way, the problem is organized and clear in your mind as well as on paper. You are less likely to make a mistake.

Multiplication and Division

In the majority of actual pharmaceutical calculations, rather than adding and subtracting fractions, we use fractions in problems involving multiplication and division. These calculations are simpler, as we do not have to have a common denominator.

Multiplying Fractions

To multiply, just multiply the top numbers of the fractions together, then multiply the bottom numbers. Then reduce the fraction.

Example: 1/4 x 1/2

Multiply the top numbers ($1 \times 1 = 1$) and bottom numbers ($4 \times 2 = 8$). Divide the top (1) by the bottom (8): the answer is 1/8.

Dividing Fractions

Division of fractions is performed a little differently. The easiest way to divide a fraction by a fraction is to flip the bottom fraction over and multiply by the top fraction.

Example: $1/4 \div 1/2$

To divide, we leave the top fraction (1/4) alone and flip over the bottom (1/2, which now becomes 2/1). Then, we multiply. Thus, 1/4 (the top) $\times$ 2/1 (the bottom, now flipped over) = 2/4. As discussed above, we want the simplest number to work with, and 2/4 can be further simplified by dividing both top and bottom by two. Then, the 2/4 becomes 1/2, which is much easier to work with (this is called reducing the fraction).

By simplifying as much as possible before doing the calculation, we not only make calculations easier but also decrease the possibility of making an error.

Working with Decimals

The modern equivalent of the fraction is the decimal. Converting fractions to decimals can make calculation easier. Decimals are commonly used with orders given in the metric system (see Chapter 11). To convert a fraction to a decimal, we simply divide the top number by the bottom and insert a point, or period, where the whole numbers end and partial numbers begin. We have all worked with decimals, and may not have realized it. Every time that you buy something and get change back, you have used the decimal system.

Decimals are based on fractions of ten. A whole number, like 1 (think of it as $1) would be expressed as ($)1.00 (100 pennies). 1/100 of a dollar is a penny, or $0.01. A dime is 1/10 of a dollar, or $0.10. 1/1000 of $1, if there was such a thing, would be 1/10 of a penny, or $0.001.

Converting Fractions to Decimals

Fractions can be easily converted to decimals just by dividing the top number of the fraction by the bottom:

Example: Convert 1/4 to a decimal.

$1 \div 4 = 0.25$. The 0 before the .25 is a placeholder that tells you there are no whole numbers. The decimal point separates the whole numbers from the fraction (decimal), which is 25 hundredths.

Use of the 0 (placeholder) before the decimal is very important. If it is not used, and the number is just written .25, there can be big problems in interpretation: the dot that you see before the 25 on the order could just be a speck of dirt on the order or computer screen, or a flaw in the paper! The order could be for 25 mg instead of 0.25 mg! Depending on the drug, that's a difference big enough to cost a patient's life. The placeholder makes it clear that the number is a decimal, and not a whole number.

Calculations with Decimals

Adding and Subtracting Decimals

Decimals are added and subtracted like regular numbers; just place the numbers above each other and calculate, being sure to keep the decimal parts separate from the whole numbers (using the decimal point).

Multiplying and Dividing Decimals

To multiply or divide decimals, we do the calculation as if no decimal was present, then place the decimal back into the answer.

Example: 1.2 × 2.5

To multiply, we first place one number above the other and multiply as usual. This give us a number—300. But, since there is one decimal place in the 1.2 and one also in the 2.5 (a total of two), we need to move the decimal place attached to the 300 over two places from the right. The answer to the problem is then 3.00. To illustrate:

1.2   (one decimal place from the right)
× 2.5   (one decimal place from the right)
3.00   (two decimal places from the right)

Remember that each time we move the decimal over one place, we are multiplying or dividing by 10. Moving the decimal one place to the **left** of the number means **dividing** by 10, while moving it one place to the **right** means **multiplying** by 10.

It is difficult to divide by a decimal without a calculator, so we make it into a whole number to divide. To divide 2.5 by 1.2, we must first multiply both numbers by 10, so that the 1.2 becomes 12 and 2.5 becomes 25. Then divide: 2.5 ÷ 1.2 = 25 ÷ 12 = 2.08.

This is a very important concept. However, you will be allowed to use calculators during the exam, so the division should be simply a matter of entering the numbers into the calculator.

Use of Algebra in Pharmaceutical Calculations

Knowledge of simple algebra is extremely useful in calculations, especially using the **ratio-proportion** method (see Chapters 14–20). Of particular use is **cross-multiplication**. If we know the relationship between two quantities, for example, milliliters and teaspoons, we can calculate another quantity that we might need. For example, say we have 100 ml of cough syrup and want to know how many one teaspoon doses are in the bottle. We set up a problem where we set the two relationships equal, and go from there:

We know that there are 5 ml per teaspoon (Chapter 11), and we have 100 ml. We set up the problem:

$$\frac{5 \text{ ml}}{1 \text{tsp}} = \frac{100 \text{ ml}}{? \text{ tsp}}$$

Then we cross multiply (using X for the amount to be calculated).

$$5 \text{ ml} \times X \text{ tsp} = 100 \text{ ml} \times 1 \text{ tsp}$$

We then try to get the X by itself, by dividing both sides of the equation by 5 ml.

$$X \text{ tsp} = \frac{100 \text{ ml} \times 1 \text{ tsp}}{5 \text{ ml}} = 20 \text{ tsp}$$

(The ml units cancel, giving the answer in tsp.)

Rounding Numbers

When a calculation produces a number that is very long and cumbersome, it is easier to round off the number. This is done by locating the last two digits at the place in the number where it should be rounded. If these two digits make a number greater than 50 (e.g., 51), round up. If it is less than 50, round down. If the number is equal to 50, then we must look at the number immediately to the left of the 50 (see example). If this number is even (2, 4, 6, 8), round the number down, if it is odd, round up.

Example: You calculate the amount to be drawn up for an injection to be 1.1256 ml. The syringe is only accurate to 0.01 ml, so you need to round off the last two numbers. Because these numbers equal 56, you round up to 1.13. If the number had been 1.1250, you would look at the number before the last two, which is a 2. The 2 is even, so you round down to 1.12.

Using Roman Numerals

A knowledge of roman numerals, both uppercase and lowercase, is necessary for the exam. In modern use, prescribers normally use lowercase roman numerals to specify the number of units of medication per dose on a written prescription. In addition, specification of amounts within the apothecary system also requires the use of roman numerals.

Roman numerals are based on a series of letters:

ss	=	1/2
I (i)	=	1
V (v)	=	5
X (x)	=	10
L (l)	=	50
C (c)	=	100
D (d)	=	500
M (m)	=	1000

When a number is written in roman numerals, the numerical values of the individual letters used should add up to the desired number (e.g., xv = 10 + 5, or 15). The roman numerals are written from left to right in order of value; for example, MCXI is 1111. If a numeral is preceded by a lesser numeral (e.g., IX), the value of the lesser numeral is subtracted from it; IX is the number 9, whereas XI is 11.

Problems for Practice

Compute the following:
1. 0.01×50
2. 0.1×25
3. 10×0.25
4. 100×0.002
5. $1/4 + 1/2$
6. $3/4 \div 1/2$
7. xxi + xiv
8. XXC + XIX

Round the following to two places:
9. 1.0035
10. 0.0255
11. 0.1550
12. 0.1450

Solutions to Problems for Practice

1–4. These all involve multiplication of decimals by a power of 10. All we need to do is to move the decimal point. Problems 1 and 2 involve multiplication by a decimal smaller than one. So, we move the decimal point to the left.

In Problem 1, (0.01 × 50.0), 0.01 has two decimal places, so we move the decimal over two places; the answer is **0.500**.

In Problem 2, 0.1 × 25.0 = **2.50**, as 0.1 only has one decimal place.

In Problems 3 and 4, we are multiplying by a power of 10, not a decimal. Since a decimal is a fraction of 10 (1/10, 1/100, etc.), and now we are multiplying by tens, we do the opposite of what we did before; we move the decimal to the right. In Problem 3, 10 × 0.25 = **2.50** as 10 has one extra decimal place. In Problem 4, 100 has two extra places (zeros), so 100 × 0.002 = **0.2**.

5. Two goes into 4 twice. The common denominator is 4. 1/2 becomes 1/2 × 2/2, or 2/4. Rewrite, and add the top numbers: 1/2 + 2/4 = **3/4**.

6. When we divide, one fraction is flipped over. Rewrite: 3/4 × 2/1 = 6/4 = **1 1/2**.

7. x = 10. Translated, these numbers become 21 + 14 (iv is 5–1 = 4). Answer: **35 (xxxv)**.

8. XX = 20. *This is subtracted* from 100 (**C**) to give 80. IX = 9, *added* to X (10), gives 19. **80 + 19 = 99 (IC)**.

9–12. We are rounding to two places, and the numbers in problems 9–12 have four places beyond the decimal. So, we take the last two places and see if they are more than, less than, or equal to 50:

In Problem 9, 35 < 50, so it rounds to 1.00.

In Problem 10, 55 > 50, so this rounds to 0.03.

In Problem 11, 50 = 50, so we look at the previous number, which is 5, an odd number. We round up to 0.16.

In Problem 12, 50 = 50, and the previous number (4) is even. We round down to 0.14.

Chapter 11

Systems of Measurement

Quick Study

(See text for full explanation.)

I. **Systems of measurement**

   A. *The household system*: teaspoons, tablespoons, cups, pints, quarts, gallons, ounces, pounds

   B. *The metric system*: liters, milliliters, microliters, kilograms, grams, milligrams, micrograms

   C. *The apothecary system*: grains, drams, scruples

II. **International units and millieqivalents**

   A. *International units*: an arbitrary conversion to the metric system which varies with a particular drug. Used to describe dosage of drugs such as insulin, penicillin, etc.

   B. *Milliequivalents*: This refers to the number of positively charged ions per liter of salt solution: *molecular weight of salt or ion ÷ ionic charge = 1 Eq*

II. **Converting units between systems**

   A. Conversion factors between systems of measurement (see table in text)

   B. Units on hand $\times \dfrac{\text{units of order}}{\text{units on hand}}$

Common Systems of Measurement

There are three basic systems of measurement which are commonly used in the pharmacy. These include the household system, metric system, and apothecary system. Of these, the metric system is the most commonly used on the order and on the manufacturer's label.

Household (or Avoirdupois) System

This is the system that the average patient would use at home. It includes *teaspoons, tablespoons, cups, pints, quarts,* and *gallons* for liquid measure, and *ounces* or *pounds* for measuring weight. The physician's order and dosage instructions may be given in the metric system and should be translated into this system of measurement which the patient can understand and use.

Metric System

This is the system used in European countries and in all disciplines of science and medicine. Here volume is measured in *liters*; 1/1000 of a liter is a *milliliter* (ml or mL), and 1/1000 of a milliliter is a *microliter* (mcl or μl). Less commonly used are *centiliters* (1/100 of a liter) and *deciliters* (1/10 of a liter). Weight is measured in *grams, milligrams,* and *micrograms* as well as the larger *kilogram*, which is 1000 grams (used in calculating dosages, see Chapter 17).

Apothecary System

This is an archaic system that is seldom used in the United States. However, a few drugs are still prescribed using apothecary weights and volumes, and you will see these measurements on the exam. In this system, volume is measured in drams and weight in grains. The scruple can be either a measure of volume or weight (see Table 11–1).

International Units and Milliequivalents

There are two other types of measurement that the technician should be familiar with. These are expressions of drug concentration. These are the international unit (U) and the milliequivalent (mEq). These are used frequently in hospital pharmacy practice and will appear on the certification exam. You will be expected to understand and use these measurements in calculations

The **international unit** system measures the amount of drug in units (IU or U). The amount of drug in milligrams varies with the drug, so unless the conversion factor is given on the manufacturer's label or referenced, conversion is not done. Examples of drugs that are measured in units are insulin, heparin, and penicillin G. The unit is used just like any other unit of measurement in calculations (e.g., mg, ml, g, etc.), so do not be intimidated by it.

A **milliequivalent (mEq)** refers to the number of positively charged ions per liter of salt solution and is normally seen on solutions of salts, such as potassium chloride (KCl). 1 Eq = the molecular weight of the salt ÷ the charge. For example, potassium has a charge of +1, so 1 Eq of KCl = (39 g + 35 g) ÷ 1 = 74 g. A 1 mEq solution would then be (74 g ÷ 1000)/L, or 74 mg per liter of solution. If the charge on the ion is more than 1, we must divide by that number; for example, calcium has a charge of +2, so 1 Eq of calcium chloride ($CaCl_2$) would be the weight of 1 calcium plus the weight of 2 chlorides, divided by 2, as calcium has a charge of +2: [40 g + 2(35 g)]/2 = 55 g, so a 1 mEq solution of calcium chloride ($CaCl_2$) would be 55 mg/L. It is not necessary to memorize molecular weights for the exam. They will be provided.

Converting Between Systems of Measurement

Converting between systems is just a matter of memorizing conversion factors and using them. Since it is easier to calculate and dispense in the metric system, conversions are usually done to and from the metric system (i.e., not from apothecary to avoirdupois, etc.) Study Table 11–1.

Table 11–1 Common Conversion Factors

(grains)	gr i	=	60 mg	
(scruples)	sc i	=	gr xx	= 1200 mg
1 lb household		=	454 g	= 16 oz
fl. oz (ℨ)	ℨ i	=	30 ml	= 8 drams
drams (ℨ)	ℨ i	=	4 ml	= 3 scruples
1 minim		=	approximately 1 gtt	
(teaspoon)	1 t	=	5 ml	
(tablespoon)	1 T	=	15 ml	
1 pint		=	16 fl oz	
1 quart		=	2 pints	≅ 1 L
1 gallon		=	4 quarts	

Note that 1 lb = 12 oz in the apothecary system but 16 oz in avoirdupois. This is irrelevant to the actual practice of pharmacy; however, these conversions may appear on the exam. If the system is not stated, assume 16 oz in a pound.

Do not confuse grains and grams. An old-fashioned way of abbreviating grams is gr. However, this is actually the abbreviation for grains. Grams should be abbreviated g, not gr. Also note that when using the apothecary system, numbers go after the unit and are expressed in roman numerals, unless the amount is less than 1/2. Example: gr v and gr ss, are correct, but gr 5 and gr 1/2 are not correct.

Converting Solid Dosage Forms Between Systems

A knowledge of these conversion factors is necessary when receiving and dispensing orders. If an order is for morphine gr iss, one must be able to quickly calculate that 1 and a half grains is 90 mg, as the morphine in stock will be measured in the more modern metric system. Additionally, one must be able to interpret the order and place instructions on the label that the patient will be able to follow. Since we do not use the metric system in the United States, if an order is dispensed with the instructions "take 5 ml bid," the technician must be able to translate this into "take 1 teaspoonful twice a day," unless a calibrated spoon or dropper is dispensed which allows the patient to measure the dose in milliliters.

To calculate the amount of medication to dispense, the first thing one should do, before attempting the calculation, is *convert* the order into the metric system. Since this system is so simple to use, attempting the calculation using any other system would be much more difficult.

Converting Units of Measure

The technician should be familiar with the following metric conversions:

1 kilogram = 1000 grams = 2.2 pounds (see Chapter 17 for explanation of kg use)

1 gram = 1000 milligrams

1 milligram = 1000 micrograms

The conversion formula is as follows:

$$\text{What you have} \times \frac{\text{What you want}}{\text{What you have}}$$

For example, say the order is for 0.5 g of drug and our stock is in milligrams. We would set up the conversion, using the values in the list above, like this:

$$0.5 \text{ g} \times \frac{1000 \text{ mg}}{\text{g}} = 500 \text{ mg.}$$ Now we can continue with the calculation.

We can do the same when converting between systems. Say our order is in grains and we need to convert to milligrams. Table 11-1 tells us that there are 60 mg/gr. So,

$$\text{gr i} \times \frac{60 \text{ mg}}{\text{gr}} = 60 \text{ mg}$$

Now that the order and stock are in the same units, our calculation can proceed.

Problem: We have an order for cough syrup, and the SIG reads: 10 ml po bid. What instructions are put on the label for the patient?

Solution: The patient will probably use a teaspoon for measure. We need to convert the instructions into teaspoons. There are 5 ml per teaspoon, so:

$$10 \text{ ml} \times \frac{1 \text{ t}}{5 \text{ ml}} = 2 \text{ t}$$

The patient should take two teaspoons of the syrup twice a day.

Problem: How many milligrams are in two scruples?

Solution: sc i = gr xx, and gr i = 60 mg, so:

Step 1. $\text{sc ii} \times \dfrac{\text{gr xx}}{\text{sc}} = \text{gr XL}$ (40 grains)

Step 2. $\dfrac{40 \text{ grains } 60 \text{ mg}}{\text{grain}} = 2400 \text{ mg}$

If we needed to, we could continue on to third and fourth steps—converting milligrams to grams, grams to kilograms, and so forth.

The key to conversion is to make sure that the units match and cancel properly. If we are looking for milligrams and have grains, for example, the grains would all have to cancel out (see above), leaving only milligrams. The units which you do want should be the only ones left, and all the others should cancel out.

Converting in Liquid Measure

Different units are used to describe a drug concentration in a measure of liquid dosage form. The most common are percent and ratio. Salt solutions are often expressed in percent: either weight/volume (*w/v*), volume/volume (*v/v*), or weight/weight (*w/w*). (See Chapter 12 for a discussion of percentages.) Drugs such as epinephrine may be expressed in a ratio. The most common expression is weight per volume.

Ratios

The concentration of some drugs (i.e., epinephrine) is expressed in the form of a ratio. This may be 1:10, 1:100, or, most commonly, 1:1000. The number on the left of the colon always means grams, and the number to the right is milliliters. Thus, 1:1000 means 1 g/1000 ml. Similarly, 1:100 = 1 g/100 ml (what is this in percent?), and 1:10 = 1 g/10 ml. Once the ratio is written out like this, it can be used in a calculation. Refer to Chapter 12 for a discussion of percentages and ratios.

Temperature Conversions

The temperature scales used in pharmacy are the fahrenheit (°F) and the centigrade or celsius (°C) scales. Traditional temperature measurements (the household scale) are in °F, and in the scientific field (and in Europe) temperature is measured in °C. Conversion may be done as follows:

$$°C = (°F - 32) \times (5/9)$$

$$°F = °C \times (9/5) + 32$$

Remember that 0°C is the freezing point of water. On the fahrenheit scale, the freezing point of water is 32°F. Thus, when we convert between the fahrenheit and centigrade scales, we must add or subtract that 32°. The temperature on the fahrenheit scale is automatically 32° more than the celsius scale (0° + 32°). Thus, when converting from fahrenheit to celsius, we subtract 32° right away before doing the actual conversion to the celsius scale. When converting the other way, from celsius to fahrenheit, we add the 32° after converting.

Remember, °F > °C ! A temperature on the fahrenheit scale is larger than that on the celsius scale, even without the 32°. You will always wind up with a smaller number when converting °F to °C and a much larger number when converting °C to °F.

Problem: If 25°C is room temperature, what is room temperature in °F ?

Solution: 25°C × (9/5) + 32 = **77°F.**

Hint: Divide the 25 by 5 first and multiply by 9

Problems for Practice

1. gr 1/4 = _____ mg
2. 5 g = _____ mg
3. 100 mcg = _____ mg
4. 1 g = _____ mcg
5. gr i ss = _____ mg
6. gr i = _____ g
7. 1 t = _____ ml
8. 5 t = _____ ml
9. 10 g = _____ kg
10. 0.5 L = _____ ml
11. gr v = _____ mg
12. How many milliliters are in 3 drams?
13. How many microliters are in 0.5 L?
14. How many teaspoons are in one tablespoon?
15. How many milliliters are in 12 ounces?
16. How many drams are in 12 ounces?
17. 100 mcg _____ mg
18. 5°C = _____ °F
19. 86°F = _____ °C
20. –5°C = _____ °F

Solutions to Problems for Practice

1. gr i = 60 mg, so gr 1/4 × 60 mg/gr = **15 mg**

2. 5 g × 1000 mg/g = **5000 mg**

3. 100 mcg × 1 mg/1000 mcg = **0.1 mg**

4. 1 g̸ × (1000 mg/g̸) × 1000 mcg/mg = **1,000,000 mcg**

5. gr iss = 1 1/2 grains, so gr iss × 60 mg/gr = **90 mg**

6. gr i = 1 grain, so g̸r i × (6̸0̸ mg/g̸r) × 1g̸/100̸0̸ mg = **0.06 g**

7. 1 t × 5 ml/t = **5 ml**

8. 5 t × 5 ml/t = **25 ml**

9. 10̸g̸ × 1 kg/100̸0̸g̸ = **0.01 kg**

10. 0.5 L̸ × 1000 ml/L̸ = **500 ml**

11. gr v is 5 grains, so g̸r v × 60 mg/g̸r = (5 × 60) mg = **300 mg**

12. 1 dram = 4 ml, so ℨ i × 4 ml/dram = **12 ml**

13. This is a two-step problem: 0.5 L × 1000 ml/L = 500 ml. 500 ml × 1000 mcl/ml = **500,000 mcl**

14. 1 t = 5 ml and 1 T = 15 ml. So, 1 T/1 t = 15 ml/5 ml = **3**

15. ℨ xii × 30 ml/ounce = (30 ml × 12) or **360 ml**

16. 360 ml are in 12 ounces, from Problem 15. ℨ i = 4 ml. 360 ml/4 ml = **90 drams**

17. 10̸0̸ mcg × 1 mg/100̸0̸ mcg = **0.1 mg**

18. We are going from little to big: use °F = °C × (9/5) + 32. Fill in the numbers: °F = 5°C × (9/5) + 32 = 32 + 9 = **41°F**

19. Use °C = (°F – 32) × (5/9). Fill in the numbers: °C = (86°F – 32) × 5/9 = 6 × 5 = **30°C.**

    Hint: Using this formula is easy, as you can do it in your head. For example, subtracting 32 from 86, we get 54. We have to multiply this by 5/9. That's the same as *dividing* the 54 by 9, and *multiplying* by **5**! From multiplication tables, we know that 9 × 6 = 54, so we just multiply **6 × 5** to get **30**

20. Use °F = °C × (9/5) + 32. Fill in the numbers:

    -5°C × (9/5) +32 and cancel:

    –5̸°C × (9/5̸) + 32 = –9 + 32 = 23°C.

    Hint: Ignore the negative sign until you add the 32 (then subtract the 9).

Chapter 12

Using Percentages and Ratios

Quick Study

(See text for full explanation.)

I.   **The percentage as a unit of measure**

    A. *Percentage = amount divided by 100:*

- *w/v* = g/100 ml
- *w/w* = g/100 g
- *v/v* = ml/100 ml

II. **Converting ratios to percentages and mg/ml**

III. **Converting from percent to grams and milligrams—filling the order**

IV. **Using alligation to combine two solutions of different percentages**

Percentage as Parts Per 100

Before we begin working with percentages, we must define what a percent is. A percent is something divided by 100. This can mean one of three things:

- g/100 ml—weight per volume [w/v], which is used in making a solution
- g/100 g—weight per weight [w/w], which might be used to make a cream or ointment
- ml/100 ml—volume per volume [v/v], which is used in mixing two fluid drugs or solutions

The principle is the same for all percents, so we will concentrate here on the most commonly used, w/v percent. When you see a % sign, always think g/100. Whenever you have a fraction or ratio that you are trying to convert to a percent, you need to convert the top number to grams and get 100 ml on the bottom. Then you have a percent. For example, if you have a solution of drug which contains 10 mg/ml, and you want to know what the percentage of drug is, you would first want to get grams on the top of your fraction (10 mg/ml). To do this, you convert the 10 milligrams to grams by moving the decimal place over three places to the left (1 g is 1000 mg—see Chapter 11). Rewrite the 10 mg/ml as 0.01 g/ml. Next, we want to get the bottom number to be 100 ml. Since we cannot just change the bottom number without doing anything to the top number, we must do the same thing to both—multiply both the top and bottom by 100, which is the same as multiplying the whole thing by one. For the bottom, 1 ml × 100 = 100 ml. Rewrite the bottom as 100 ml. The top number would become 0.01 g × 100 = 1 g. Now we have converted the 10 mg/ml into 1 g/100 ml, which is 1%.

When changing a fraction to a percent, always think g/100 ml. To change a percent to a fraction, do the opposite—express the percent as grams (or milligrams) per 100 ml and simplify (this usually works best if we turn the grams into milligrams and then divide by 100, to get mg/ml).

Example: You have 1 g of drug in 50 ml of solution. What is the percent of the solution?

Solution: Your ratio is 1 g/50 ml. You want g/100 ml. You have grams on the top of the ratio already, so leave that. You now need to have 100 ml on the bottom to get a percent. So you multiply the 50 ml on the bottom by 2. Since you did that, you must also multiply the top number by 2 (so you are multiplying the whole thing by 2/2, which is 1).

$$1 \text{ g/50 ml} \times 2/2 = 2 \text{ g/100 ml.}$$

Your solution is 2%.

What happens if a solution of drug is in percent and the order is in milligrams? You can easily convert a percentage solution into mg/ml in order to fill a prescription.

Example: You have a solution of 1% lidocaine. What is the concentration in mg/ml?

Solution: 1% = 1 g/100 ml. We want mg, so convert the 1 g to 1000 mg. Rewrite: 1000 mg/100 ml, and cancel. The solution is 10 mg/ml. Now you can accurately draw up an order for 2 mg of lidocaine from an ampule of 1% lidocaine solution (see Chapter 15).

You can take the problem one step further and ask: "How many mg are in 10 ml of this solution?" (Say that you have 10 ml of 1% lidocaine, and need a certain amount to fill an order. You want to see if you have enough.) You have previously calculated that the 1% lidocaine contained 10 mg of lidocaine/ml. To determine the amount of drug contained in a particular volume (10 ml, in this case), you simply multiply:

Remember: Concentration of drug ×
volume of solution = **amount** of drug

In 10 ml of 1% lidocaine, we have 10 ml × 10 mg/ml = 100 mg of drug available for dispensing.

Using Alligation

Now we will address how to make a percentage solution when two solutions of different concentrations are available. For this calculation, we can use a method called **alligation**. This method only works with two solutions that have different percentages of drug, when we want to make a solution with a third percentage of drug.

For example, say you have a 20% solution and a 5% solution of calcium gluconate in stock, but you need a 10% solution. How can you mix these two solutions together to get a 10% solution?

First make a chart, as follows:

20%	⇒	5 parts
	10%	
5%	⇒	10 parts

Note that the more concentrated solution (20% stock) is in the upper left corner, and the less concentrated solution (5% stock) is in the lower left corner. The solution that you are trying to make (10%) goes in the middle. The concentration of the solution that you are trying to make (in this case the 10% solution) must have a concentration intermediate between the two stock solutions (5% solution and the 20% solution). To figure out how much of each stock solution that you have to mix together to get the 10% solution, simply subtract the numbers diagonally: 20 − 10 (= **10**), and 10 − 5 (= **5**). Now look *across* the chart (see arrows). The 5 is on the same line as the 20%, so you need to have *five* parts of the 20% solution. The 10 is on the same line as the 5%, so you need *ten* parts of the 5% solution to mix with the 20% solution.

How much is a "part"? This depends on how much of the 10% solution that you need to make: For example, let's say that you need to make 150 ml of the 10% solution. From the chart, you need *five* parts of the 20% solution and *ten* parts of the 5% solution, which is *fifteen* parts total. You need to make 150 ml total. Thus, the volume of one part is 150 ml/15 parts = 10 ml/part. Therefore, we add 100 ml (10 parts × 10 ml/part) of the 5% solution, and 50 ml of the 20% solution (5 parts × 10 ml/part) to make 150 ml of the 10% solution:

5 parts of the 20% solution

+10 parts of the 5% solution
_____

15 parts total

150 ml needed ÷ 15 parts total =

10 ml/part

10 parts of 5% solution = 10 parts × 10 ml/part = **100 ml**

5 parts of 20% solution = 5 parts × 10 ml/part = **50 ml**

To summarize:

- Fill in the alligation chart properly, with the desired concentration in the middle space.
- Subtract the numbers diagonally.
- Look across the top and bottom of the chart to determine the relative amounts of each solution to add together (number of parts of each).
- Add the number of parts together.
- Divide the desired volume of solution that you wish to make by the total number of parts of both solutions, to determine the amount of volume per part.
- Mix the two solutions together in the appropriate volumes.

Using Drug Concentrations Expressed as a Ratio

You will need to know how to convert a ratio to a percentage, and to convert dosage amounts from a ratio. As explained in Chapter 11, a ratio is two numbers separated by a colon (e.g., 1:10, 1:100, or 1:1000). The number on the left of the colon is always in grams, and the number to the right is in milliliters. Thus, a 1:1000 solution of drug would have a concentration of 1g of drug per 1000 ml. Similarly, 1:100 solution would have 1 g drug per 100 ml and so on. Once the ratio is written out as grams per unit of volume, it can be used in the conversion calculation.

Converting Dosages From a Ratio

To use a stock concentration which is expressed in a ratio to fill an order, first write the ratio as grams/volume in milliliters. Then proceed with the calculation. It might be helpful for you to memorize the three most commonly encountered ratios in terms of mg/ml. These are as follows:

1:1000 = 1 mg/ml, 1:100 = 10 mg/ml and 1:10 = 100 mg/ml

Problem: Your order is for 1 mg of epinephrine, and the available stock is a 1:100 solution. What volume is dispensed?

Solution:

Step 1: Write down both order and stock. Recall that 1:100 is 1 g/100 ml. The order is in mg, so convert the g to mg:

1 g̸ × 1000 mg/g̸ = 1000 mg. The 1 g/100 ml now becomes 1000 mg/100 ml. Cancel zeros, and 1000 mg/100 ml becomes 10 mg/ml.

Step 2: Calculate the amount dispensed (Use either method. I will use order ÷ stock). You dispense 0.1 ml of epinephrine to fill the order.

$$\frac{1\ mg}{10\ mg/ml} = 0.1\ ml$$

You may also see a problem on the exam which will ask you to calculate the dose received by the patient. Calculate this as follows:

Problem: You dispense a bolus injection of 0.5 ml of a 1:1000 solution of epinephrine. Calculate the dose of epinephrine which the patient will receive.

Solution:

Step 1: Convert the stock to mg/ml: 1 g/1000 ml = 1000 mg/1000 ml = 1 mg/ml.

Step 2: Set up the problem so that the units cancel, leaving you with a dose in mg

0.5 m̸l̸ × 1 mg/m̸l̸ = **0.5 mg**

Converting From a Ratio to a Percentage

To convert from a ratio to a percentage, the calculation is easy. Suppose we want to determine the percentage of drug in a 1:100 solution. First, always write out the ratio: 1:100 = 1 g/100 ml. By definition, a 1% solution is 1 g/100 ml. Therefore, a 1:100 solution is 1%.

Problems for Practice

1. Express 1:1000 in mg/ml.

2. An opthalmic solution contains 1% drug solution. If a patient uses 0.2 ml of drug per eye, what is the dose of drug being placed in each eye?

3. You have 5 ml of a 2% solution and need to dispense a 5 mg dose. How many doses are in the bottle?

4. A suppository contains 5% zinc oxide. How much zinc oxide is contained in a 5 g suppository?

5. A 5 g suppository contains 0.5% phenylephrine and 20% zinc oxide as the active ingredients. What percentage of the active ingredients is made up by the phenylephrine?

6. You need 80 ml of a 2% solution of boric acid. You have a 1% solution, and a 5% solution in stock. How do you make the 2% solution?

7. A procedure for making cortizone cream states that the cream contains 200 mg of cortizone per milliliter of cream. What is the percentage of the cortizone?

8. You are making lactated Ringer's solution. The procedure calls for 20 g of lactic acid per liter. What is the percentage of lactic acid?

9. 500 ml of cream contains 5 g menthol. What is the percentage of menthol?

10. How many grams of zinc chloride are needed to make 1500 ml of a 2% solution?

11. How many mg are in 15 ml of a 5% solution?

12. A solution contains 2 g of drug per 25 ml of solution. What is the percentage of drug in the solution?

13. You have 5 g of sodium chloride. How much saline (0.9%) can you make?

14. What is the concentration in mg/ml of a 7% solution?

15. Express 2% in terms of a ratio.

16. You need to make 100 ml of a 5% solution. You have 60 ml of a 10% solution and 50 ml of a 2% solution. Can you fill the order?

17. How many milligrams of cortizone are in 5 g of a 1% cortizone cream?

18. A solution of drug is 50 mg/ml. What is the percentage of drug?

19. How many mg of drug are in 5 ml of a 1:100 solution?

Solutions to Problems for Practice

1. 1:1000 is 1 gram/1000 ml. So, since 1 g = 1000 mg, 1:1000 is also 1000 mg/1000 ml = **1 mg/ml.** It would be wise to memorize this one, as it comes up often.

2. This is really only a simple conversion problem. 1% is 1 g/100 ml of solution:

    0.2 ~~ml~~ /eye × 1 g/100 ~~ml~~ = 0.002 g. It would be easier to express this in mg—
    0.002 g × 1000 mg/g = **2 mg/dose** in each eye.

3. The question here is how many milligrams are in the bottle? 2% = 2 g/100 ml = 2000 mg/100 ml. 5 ~~ml~~ × 2000 mg/100 ~~ml~~ = 100 mg. The question asks how many 50 mg doses are in the bottle: 100 mg/bottle ÷ 5 mg/dose = **20 doses.**

4. This is a weight per weight (w/w) percent problem. 5% is now 5 g/100 g. The problem is solved in the same way as before:

    5 ~~g~~ × 5 g/100 ~~g~~ = 25/100 g or **0.25 g** (250 mg).

5. This problem is a bit more complicated. If the suppository weighs 5 g, then:
    *   the amount of phenylephrine is 0.5% of 5 g, or 5 g × 0.5 g/100 g = 0.025 g = 25 mg.
    *   the amount of zinc oxide is 20% of 5 g, or 1 g.
    *   the total amount of the active ingredients is 1 g + 0.025 g = 1.025 g.

    The question asks what percent of the active ingredients is made up of phenylephrine. If the phenylephrine is 0.025 g, and the total is 1.025 g, we can determine a percentage by dividing: (0.025 g ÷ 1.025 g) × 100% = **2.4%.**

6. We can use alligation for this problem. First we make the chart:

1%	⇒	3 parts
	2%	
5%	⇒	1 part

    The solutions in stock are 1% and 5%, so these are put on the left. You want a 2% solution, so 2% goes in the middle. You subtract 5–2 to get 3 on the top and 2–1 to get 1 on the bottom. These numbers refer to the relative amounts of the two solutions used. According to the chart above, you need one part of the 5% solution to three parts of the 1% solution. The volume of a part is variable, depending on how much volume you need. Since you need 80 ml total, you determine how much a part is by dividing 80 ml by 4 (1 part + 3 parts, from the chart). One part = 80/4 or 20 ml. *Therefore, the solution to the problem is to mix 20 ml of the 5% solution (1 part × 20 ml) with 60 ml (3 parts × 20 ml) of the 1% solution.*

7. Percentage is in g/100 ml, so you need to get the ratio of cortizone to cream in g/100 ml:

    200 mg cortizone × 1 g/1000 mg = 0.2 g cortizone.

    If there are 200 mg cortizone (0.2 g) per 1 ml of cream, there must be:

    0.2 g × 100 = 20 g per 1 ml × 100 = 100 ml of cream.

    20 g/100 ml = **20%.**

8. 20 g/1000 ml (1 L) is given in the problem. Simply cancel zeros: 2~~0~~ g/100~~0~~ ml = 2 g/100 ml. The answer is **2%.**

9. 5 g/500 ml = 1 g/100 ml. Answer: **1%.**

10. A 2% solution is 2 g/100 ml. You need 1500 ml, so you must multiply:

$$2 \text{ g}/100 \text{ ml} \times 1500 \text{ ml} = \textbf{30 g.}$$

11. 5% = 5 g/100 ml. 5 g = 5000 mg, so 5% = 5000 mg/100 ml.

    Do the problem: 15 ml × 5000 mg/100 ml = **750mg.**

12. You have 2 g/25 ml. To have percent, you need g/100 ml. So, you multiply by 4/4:

$$2 \text{ g}/25 \text{ ml} \times 4/4 = 8 \text{ g}/100 \text{ ml} = \textbf{8\%.}$$

13. The easiest way to do this one is by ratio/proportion (Chapter 14). However, you can also do the problem using simple division and multiplication: saline is 0.9 g of sodium chloride per 100 ml (0.9%). If you divide your 5 g by 0.9 g/100 ml, you can determine the volume that you can make: (5 g/0.9 g) × 100 ml = **555.6 ml** (see Division by Fractions, Chapter 10).

14. 7% is 7 g/100 ml. Convert the 7 g to mg:

$$7 \text{ g} \times 1000 \text{ mg}/\text{g} = 7000 \text{ mg.}$$

    Rewrite and cancel:

$$7000 \text{ mg}/100 \text{ ml} = \textbf{70 mg/ml}$$

15. 2% = 2 g/100ml = 2000 mg/100 ml = **20 mg/ml.**

16. This problem would require alligation. Fill in the chart:

10%	⇒	3 parts
	5%	
2%	⇒	5 parts

    According to the chart, you would need 3 parts of the 10% solution and 5 parts of the 2% solution. That makes 8 parts, which must equal 100 ml as stated by the problem. 100 ml/8 parts = 12.5 ml/part. You would then need 3 parts × 12.5 ml = 37.5 ml of the 10%, and 5 parts × 12.5 ml = 62.5 ml of the 2% solution. You have 60 ml of the 10% and need only 37.5 ml, but you need 62.5 ml of the 2% and have only 50 ml. The answer: **No,** you cannot make the solution.

17. 5 g cream × 1 g of cortizone/100 g cream = 0.05 g cortizone.
    0.05 g cortizone × 1000 mg/g = **50 mg.**

    You could also do this problem by ratio and proportion: since 1 g = 1000 mg, and the percentage of cortizone in the cream is 1%

$$\frac{1000 \text{ mg cortizone}}{100 \text{g cream}} = \frac{X}{5 \text{ g cream}}$$

18. 5% = 5g/100 ml. A ratio has grams on the left and ml on the right. So, 5% = 5:100.

19. 1:100 = 1 g/100 ml = 1000 mg/100 ml = 10mg/ml

$$5 \text{ml} \times 10 \text{mg/ml} = \textbf{50mg.}$$

Chapter 13

Measuring Equipment

Quick Study

(See text for full explanation.)

I. **Measurement of solutions**

    A. *Small volumes*:

- Use of a *calibrated* syringe, dosage cup, or dropper
- Proper use of syringes calibrated in international units (i.e., insulin syringes)

    B. *Larger volumes: graduated cylinder*

    C. The *size* of any measuring container and *calibrations should be appropriate to the volume* to be measured

II. **Measurement of solid materials—bulk compounding and bulk manufacturing**

    A. Torsion balance

    B. Double pan balance

    C. Prescription balance

III. **Pitfalls to inaccurate measurement**

    A. The *effect* of temperature on the accuracy of measurement

    B. Failure to use *clean equipment*

    C. Failure to read the volume measurement at the appropriate place (i.e., syringe plunger, meniscus of cylinder)

    D. Use of *improper size or calibration* of measuring equipment

There are two types of measurement that we need to be concerned with: solid measurement, which would be used in bulk compounding, for example, and liquid measurement. Because liquid measurement is the most common, we will begin the discussion here.

Liquid Measurement

Solutions and suspensions must be measured using accurate devices. For small volumes (less than 10 ml), a syringe may be used for accurate measure. For larger volumes (greater than 10 ml), a **graduated cylinder** should be used.

The measuring device used to dispense a liquid of any type should be the closest possible size to the volume being measured. In general, measuring devices for liquids are considered to be accurate to 20% of their volume. Graduations and markings are less detailed on larger devices, however, so the accuracy of measurement becomes less. For example, if an order calls for 10 ml of a solution for oral dosage, a graduated cylinder which holds 100 ml should not be used. If possible, a 10 ml cylinder or syringe should be used. If these are not available, the size of device closest to the volume being measured should be chosen (i.e., a 20 ml syringe or 25 ml graduated cylinder).

Solutions should also be measured all at once. Each time a solution is measured in a device, some solution clings to the inside when it is emptied. Syringes have a rubber plunger that fits closely to the sides of the barrel and helps to scrape off any material sticking to the sides, so less drug remains on the plastic. Even so, it is not necessarily a good practice to use any device more than once for measuring.

The temperature of the solution or of the work area will also affect the accuracy of measurements. When liquids are warm, they expand and take up more volume. When cooled, they contract, and less volume will be measured. Thus, if we are in a warm room while measuring, the patient will actually get less drug, as the volume which we measured was deceptively expanded—instead of dispensing 10 ml of solution (containing 100 mg of drug, we actually dispensed only 9.8 ml (98 mg of drug), but it had expanded to look like 10 ml, due to the warm temperature. The patient will be underdosed.

In the same way, if a solution is taken from the refrigerator, the volume measured will appear smaller and, unless the medication is allowed to warm to room temperature before measuring, the patient will get a solution of drug that is slightly more concentrated than what is desired. Temperature is also important in weight measurements (see below).

Devices for Measuring Liquids

There are essentially two types of measuring devices for liquids: the graduated cylinder, which is used to measure and dispense liquids intended for oral dosage, and the syringe, which is used to measure and dispense liquids intended for parenteral dosage.

Devices used by the patient for measure are the calibrated dropper, calibrated spoon, oral syringe, and dosage cup. These devices are not used for dispensing but allow the patient or caregiver to more accurately measure the medication. For example, if the instructions for the medication are to place one drop in each eye, the patient could come up with any number of droppers, all of which dispense a different size of drop (and thus a different dosage of drug than was prescribed). A *calibrated* dropper has markings to show how much drug solution is actually being given, as opposed to a household "eye dropper," which has no calibrations and dispenses an unknown amount of drug per drop. The same problem applies to a spoon. I have seen "teaspoons" that hold about two ml, as well as "tablespoons" that hold about 1 oz! Using a *calibrated* spoon to administer medication ensures correct dosing. These spoons are often adjustable, to administer different amounts if necessary, and thus can be used with more than one prescription.

The oral syringe and dosage cup are also used for oral dosing. The oral syringe may look like a syringe for parenteral administration (it has no needle attachment, which precludes the nurse or technician from grabbing the wrong syringe by mistake and administering an oral medication by injection), or it may simply be a fat plastic syringe with a rubber squeeze bulb at the top, such as the kind commonly sold in drug stores. Again, the calibrations, which are in milliliters, make accurate dosing easier (no conversion is necessary).

The dosage cup is plastic, and holds one ounce (30 ml). It normally has markings on the sides for measurement in all three systems: drams, milliliters, and (one) ounce. The smallest amount that can be accurately measured in a dosage cup is one dram (4 ml). The measurements on a dosage cup are really not very accurate; they are designed for things like cough syrups, where an overdose or underdose of a milliliter or two is not critical. None of the calibrated equipment for oral dosage is really very accurate—not like a syringe for parenteral injection, which must be very accurate. One needs to bear in mind that the patient, when measuring the drug, is not going to be very fastidious about measuring and may not even be able to see clearly!

Dispensing Large Volumes of Liquid—The Graduated Cylinder

When dispensing a large volume of a liquid for oral use, a graduated cylinder is normally used. This is a glass or plastic cylinder that has graduations, or markings for measurement, on the sides (Figure 13–1). When using a plastic cylinder, you may simply fill the cylinder to the appropriate mark and read the correct volume from the marking scale. However, when using a glass cylinder, measurement is a little more complicated. In a plastic cylinder, the top of the liquid appears as a straight line and is easy to read. However, in a glass cylinder, the light from the room refracts off of the glass and causes an optical illusion that the surface of the liquid inside the cylinder is curved. This "curved" portion is called the **meniscus**. When reading the correct volume from a glass cylinder, one must look not at the top of the liquid but at the bottom of the curved part (meniscus). Graduated cylinders can be calibrated, if necessary, by filling the cylinder with an amount of water and weighing it; 1 ml of water should weigh 1 g at 25°C.

Figure 13-1   The graduated cylinder and meniscus

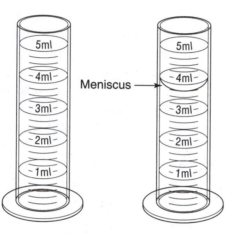

Accurately Dispensing Small Volumes—The Syringe

The syringe for injection is made of sterile plastic and is made to accommodate a needle. In contrast the oral syringe, which is not sterile, does not accommodate a needle. It is made for oral dosing, as discussed previously. The sterile syringe is calibrated, with the type of calibrations depending on the size of the syringe: a 0.5 ml syringe is calibrated in increments of 0.005 ml, a 1 ml syringe (tuberculin, or TB syringe) in 0.01 ml, and the larger sizes (3, 5, and 10 ml) in 0.1 ml (see Figure 13–2). A syringe is only accurate to the smallest calibration. When a syringe is used, the amount of solution drawn up is measured by the first black line (nearest the plunger tip) made by the side of the plunger, not the rubber cone that extends into the solution (see Figure 13–2). Again, solutions should be as close to room temperature as possible (without harming the drug) before measuring, to avoid errors in measurement.

Insulin Syringes

Syringes intended for the administration of insulin are used only for that purpose. They are calibrated in **international units**, specific to the con-

Figure 13-2   A 3 cc syringe

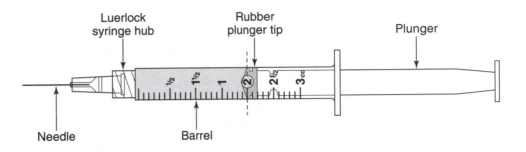

centration of normal insulin only. They may not be used with any other drug which might be measured in units (e.g., heparin, streptomycin, penicillin), as the amount of drug per unit varies with the drug. Insulin syringes are to be used for the measurement of insulin only. The needle on the syringe is permanently attached and is a 30 gauge needle (abbreviated on the packaging as "30G"; you may also see "ga" used, which is an older abbreviation). This needle is very fine and easily bent. (See Chapter 17 for a discussion of needles.) *Note that 100 units of normal insulin is equivalent to 1 ml volume.* This conversion is important, because, if no insulin syringes are available, a tuberculin (1 ml) syringe may be used as follows: the amount of insulin dispensed can be calculated by dividing the order by 100 U/ml (normal insulin) to obtain the amount to dispense in milliliters. The insulin can then be dispensed in a tuberculin (1 ml) syringe with a 30 g needle or, in an emergency, a standard 25 g or 27 g needle.

Measuring Solids

Measuring devices are normally not used to dispense a solid drug (e.g., tablet, capsule) directly. However, if a solution or semisolid dosage form is to be compounded (a procedure that the technician may legally perform if written instructions exist—see Chapter 21), a weight scale may be used. To accurately weigh a gram of material or more, there are at least two methods. Weighing very small amounts (1 mg or less) cannot be done by either of these methods—this requires a special type of scale, which is very expensive and difficult to use.

To weigh large quantities of material, such as that required to make a solution, a **torsion balance** or **solution balance** may be used. This balance has only one weighing pan, which hangs at the end of the scale, and is not very sensitive (thus it could not be used to weigh small quantities).

Another piece of equipment designed for weighing large quantities is the **double-pan balance**. It is the oldest of the devices used for weighing large quantities (grams and kilograms). This device balances (or hangs) two pans opposite each other and works on the principle of gravity. The material to be weighed is placed on one pan. On the other is placed one or more carefully calibrated counterweights. When the two pans balance, the weight of the material is equal to the weight of the counterweights, and the weight of the material can be determined (each counterweight weighs a specific amount, which is printed on it).

A similar system used to weigh much smaller quantities is the **prescription balance**. This is a more sensitive instrument, weighing as little as 5 or 6 mg accurately, but it cannot weigh large quantities; the largest amount weighed is about 100 to 120 g.

When these instruments are used to weigh material, the positions of the material being weighed and the counterweights on the surface of the pans are critical for accurate measurement; both the material to be weighed and the counterweights must be placed exactly in the middle of the weighing pan. If they are not, the weights obtained for the material will not be accurate, because the pan will list to one side. Also, the counterweights should not be touched, as skin oil from the fingers adds weight. Forceps or padded tweezers should always be used to carefully handle the weights.

As with liquid measurement, *temperature is critical in weight measurements*. With solid measurements, however, the expansion of the material with temperature is not the problem. A difference in the temperature of the material in relation to the scale will actually change the weight measurement. If the material to be weighed is warm, it will warm the air around it, creating air currents that surround the material and rise, slightly lifting the material off of the pan and causing the weight reading to be lower than it really is. The effect is very slight but can make a big difference in the weight measurement. As the material cools, more of the material will rest on the pan and the weight will then appear to increase, so that if it is weighed several times, the weights will vary as the material cools (if your scale is cold, and the material that you are weighing is at room temperature, you may have the same effect). Weighing any material when warm or cold will result in an inaccurately prepared drug product.

Questions for Review

1. To measure 15 ml of cough syrup, a ____ should be used.
   1. 10 ml graduated cylinder, used twice
   2. 10 ml syringe, used twice
   3. 20 ml graduated cylinder
   4. 50 ml graduated cylinder

2. You dispense 10 ml of a suspension for oral dosing, from the refrigerator. As a result, the patient could:
   1. be overdosed.
   2. be underdosed.
   3. receive the correct dose.
   4. have an anaphylactic reaction to the drug.

3. In order to be sure that an accurate amount of opthalmic solution is placed into the eye, the patient should be provided with:
   1. a dosage cup.
   2. an eye dropper.
   3. a calibrated dropper.
   4. a syringe.

4. When a graduated cylinder made of glass is used, an accurate reading of the amount of fluid measured would be made by looking at the:
   1. top of the fluid in the cylinder.
   2. sides of the meniscus.
   3. bottom of the meniscus.
   4. marking on the cylinder that is closest to the fluid.

5. At 25° C, 1 ml of water weighs:
   1. 10 mg.
   2. 5 g.
   3. 100 mg.
   4. 1 g.

6. When a double pan balance is used to weigh material for compounding, the:
   1. sample and weights should be placed in the middle of their pans.
   2. weights should not be touched.
   3. sample to be weighed should not be less than the total of the counterweights.
   4. all of the above are true.

7. A cream compounded by the technician that was supposed to contain 2% cortisone was found to contain only 1.8% cortizone. A probable explanation might be that:
   1. the technician handled the counterweights when weighing.
   2. the cortizone was cooler than the scale.
   3. the cortizone was contaminated, from the supplier.
   4. the cortizone was weighed on the wrong type of scale.

Solutions to Questions for Review

1. You want to measure the liquid in a device that is of the closest possible size. The best answer would be **3**, a 20 ml graduated cylinder, as it is closest to 15 ml.

2. A solution taken from the refrigerator will be condensed, due to the cold. When the solution is measured cold and then allowed to warm to room temperature, it will expand. The patient may receive too much drug and may be overdosed. The correct answer is **1.**

3. A household eye dropper is not calibrated; the drop size varies from dropper to dropper. To receive an accurate dose of medication, the patient would need to receive a dropper that is calibrated for the medication. A syringe is calibrated but would be awkward to use. The correct answer is **3**.

4. A glass cylinder refracts light and makes the top of the solution appear curved (the meniscus). Thus, you would want to look at the markings on the cylinder where the bottom of the meniscus falls. The correct answer is **3**.

5. The weight of water at 25° C is important for calibration of measuring equipment. Water weighs 1 g/ml at 25° C. The correct answer is **4**.

6. All of the statements are true. The correct answer is **4**.

7. If the calculations were performed correctly and the scale was used correctly, it is possible that there was a temperature difference between the cortizone and the scale. The drug scale may have been in a cold room. The correct answer is **2**.

Chapter 14

Conversion of Solid Dosage Forms

Quick Study

(See text for full explanation.)

I. **Converting the order to match the available stock in terms of weight of drug per dose**
   A. *Converting between units* to match order to the available stock
   B. *Order ÷ stock = amount dispensed*
   C. *Using the ratio/proportion method*

Pharmacies stock only a limited supply of drugs and drug dosage forms, as compared to what is available. Perhaps one strength of a particular drug tablet is more popular than another, so the pharmacy stocks only that strength which is most commonly ordered. An order, however, is made by a prescriber who does not necessarily have much knowledge of the pharmacy or its formulary. So, it is necessary, on occasion, to *convert* the order to match the stock available. This can only be done if the dosage form is appropriate to the conversion — scored tablets, for example. In order to convert an order, we must follow three steps:

1. Make sure that the units (e.g., mg, g) of both the order and stock match. If they do not, convert one to match the other. (Which one is converted really makes no difference. I prefer converting the order to match the stock.)

2. Divide the order by the available stock (or use the ratio/proportion method, as discussed below) to obtain the amount dispensed.

3. Make sure that your answer is within your range of measurements. If not, you may not be able to fill the order. For example, if you calculate that ten tablets must be dispensed from your stock per dose, or that 10 ml must be dispensed for an IM injection, the conversions

are unacceptable, and you must use a stock with a higher dosage strength.

Let's do some problems.

Problem: You have an order for Lasix tabs, 80 mg bid #30. The pharmacy has only 40 mg tablets.

Solution: There are at least two ways to do this type of problem. The first is to divide the order by the stock, to get the number of tablets dispensed. **Remember:** Order ÷ Stock = amount dispensed per dose.

Step 1:   *Write down the information which you have.* (If you are faced with a "story" problem on the exam, this is especially useful; you must first ask yourself what the question is asking—what does the examiner want to know. Then think of how you would figure it out, and go to the problem and extract the appropriate information. That way, you will not be confused by extra information that may be given in the problem.)

Order = 80 mg tablets, stock available = 40 mg tablets.

Step 2:   Divide the order by the stock.

80 mg/dose ÷ 40 mg/tablet = 2 tablets dispensed per dose.

Answer: Since the order is for 30 of the 80 mg tablets, we dispense 30×2, or 60 tablets of the 40 mg strength.

A second and very valuable way to do this type of calculation is by the *ratio/proportion* method. This method is very helpful, particularly for liquid dosage conversions (see Chapters 15 and 16). In this method, we make a *ratio* of the order and a ratio of the stock and set them equal, solving algebraically, like we did in Chapter 10:

Example: Order: $\dfrac{80 \text{ mg}}{1 \text{ dose}}$ = Stock: $\dfrac{40 \text{ mg}}{1 \text{ tablet}}$

Cross multiply: 80 mg × 1 tablet = 1 dose × 40 mg

Now, we want to get the dose by itself to find out how much it is. So, we divide both sides by 40 mg to find out how much to dispense, per dose.

$$\frac{80 \text{ mg} \times 1 \text{ tablet}}{40 \text{ mg}} = \frac{40 \text{ mg} \times 1 \text{ dose}}{40 \text{ mg}}$$

The 40 mg values cancel, and the dose = 80/40 = 2 tablets/dose.

Problem: Your order is for digoxin tablets, 0.25 mg. You have 0.5 mg tabs in stock.

Solution: $\dfrac{\text{Order}}{\text{Stock}} = \dfrac{0.25 \text{ mg/dose}}{0.5 \text{ mg/tab}} = 1/2$ tablet per dose

As discussed previously, whenever you work with a number problem, you must make sure that the *units* assigned to the numbers (e.g., g, mg, gr, etc.) are the same before attempting the problem. In other words, if your order is in milligrams and your stock is in grams, you must first convert either the stock to milligrams or the order to grams before beginning the calculation, such as in the following example.

Problem: Your order is for ampicillin, 0.5 g per dose. The pharmacy stocks ampicillin in 250 mg capsules.

Solution: First, recalling that there are 1000 mg/g, convert the 0.5 g to mg, to match the stock.

$$0.5 \cancel{g} \times \frac{1000 \text{ mg}}{1 \cancel{g}} = 500 \text{ mg}$$

Then, do the calculation:

Order ÷ stock = 500 mg ÷ 250 mg/capsule = 2 capsules/dose

Be aware, however, that the calculation could not be done the opposite way! Since capsules are not scored and cannot be easily broken in half, an order for 250 mg could not be filled if the pharmacy stocked only 500 mg capsules.

Converting Between Measurement Systems

Although the apothecary system is rather archaic, you may still receive orders signed in grains or drams (scruples and minims are not used in practice; however, they may appear on the exam). Know how to convert between the metric and apothecary systems (see Chapter 11 for review).

Problem: You have an order for morphine gr 1/4 po bid prn. You have 30 mg tablets in stock (scored in fourths). What do you dispense? (**Remember:** convert the units first, before continuing with the problem.)

Solution: One dose is 1/4 grain. Recall that gr i is 60 mg. First, convert the units; in this case, I would convert grains to milligrams, since they are easier to work with:

$$1/4 \cancel{\text{grain}} \times \frac{60 \text{ mg}}{\cancel{\text{grain}}} = 15 \text{ mg}$$

Then, do the calculation:

$$\frac{15 \text{ mg}}{30 \text{ mg}} = 1/2 \text{ tablet per dose.}$$

Problem: You have an order for penicillin G, 200,000 U q4h. You have 400,000 U strength tablets in stock.

Solution: $\dfrac{200,000 \cancel{U}}{400,000 \cancel{U}/\text{tablet}} = 1/2 \text{ tablet}$

Do not let the various units confuse you! As long as the units match between order and stock, the calculation can be done. If you encounter international units and you need to convert, the conversion factor should be on the product label—for instance, 250 mg of Penicillin G is 400,000 U.

Problems for Practice

Calculate the amount of tablets dispensed, per dose, given the following:

1. You have an order for Decadron 1.5 mg po bid. You have 750 mcg tabs in stock.
2. Your order is for prednisolone 0.05 g po q6h. You have 25 mg tabs in stock.
3. Your order is for digoxin 125 mcg po qd. Your stock is 0.25 mg tabs, scored in four.
4. Your order is for morphine gr ss. Your stock is 30 mg tabs.
5. Your order is for furosemide 80 mg bid. You have 40 mg Lasix tabs in stock.
    (a) Dispense one dose.
    (b) Dispense a unit dose.
6. Your order is for phenytoin 50 mg tid. You have Dilantin, 100 mg tabs (scored).
    (a) Dispense one dose.
    (b) Dispense a unit dose.
7. Your order is for Orinase, 250 mg. Your stock is 0.5 g tablets (scored).
8. Your order is for penicillin, 600,000 U po. You have 250 mg tabs in stock. The label says that one 250 mg tablet contains 400,000 U. The tablets are scored in half.
9. You have an order for Synthroid 0.1 mg. You have 50 mcg tablets available.
10. Your order is for aspirin gr v. You have 300 mg tablets available.
11. Your order is for morphine gr iss. You have 30 mg tablets in stock.
12. Your order is for KCl, 20 mEq. You have 10 mEq tablets in stock.
13. Your order is for morphine gr 1/4. You have 30 mg tablets in stock, scored in fourths.
14. You have a vial containing 500 mg of morphine. How many doses of gr iss can be filled from the bottle?
15. You have an order for Motrin 400 mg bid. You have 800 mg tablets in stock.

Solutions to Problems for Practice

1. First, convert the order to match the stock:

    $$1.5 \text{ mg} \times 1000 \text{ mcg/mg} = 1500 \text{ mcg}.$$

    Do the problem:

    $$\text{order} \div \text{stock} = 1500 \text{ mcg} \div 750 \text{ mcg/tablet} = \textbf{2 tablets dispensed.}$$

2. First, convert:

    $$0.05 \text{ g} \times 1000 \text{ mg/g} = 50.0 \text{ mg}.$$

    Do the problem:

    $$50.0 \text{ mg} \div 25 = \textbf{2 tablets per dose dispensed.}$$

3. First, convert:

    $$125 \text{ mcg} \times 1 \text{ mg/1000 mcg} = 0.125 \text{ mg/dose}.$$

    Do the problem:

    $$0.125 \text{ mg} \div 0.25 \text{ mg/tablet} = \textbf{1/2 tablet per dose dispensed}.$$

4. First, convert:

    $$\text{gr ss} = 1/2 \text{ grain. } 1/2 \text{ gr} \times 60 \text{ mg/gr} = 30 \text{ mg}.$$

    Do the problem:

    $$30 \text{ mg} \div 30 \text{ mg/tablet} = \textbf{1 tablet dispensed per dose.}$$

5. No conversion necessary:

    $$80 \text{ mg} \div 40 \text{ mg/tablet} = \textbf{2 tablets per dose.}$$

    A *unit* dose is the dose × number of doses per day = 2 tablets × 2 doses/day = **4 tablets.**

6. No conversion necessary. 50 mg ÷ 100 mg/tablet = **1/2 tablet per dose.**

    A *unit* dose would be 1/2 tablet/dose × three doses/day = **1.5 tablets.**

7. First, convert:

    $$250 \text{ mg} \times 1 \text{ g/1000 mg} = 0.25 \text{ g}.$$

    Do the problem:

    $$0.25 \text{ g} \div 0.5 \text{ g/dose} = \textbf{1/2 tablet per dose.}$$

8. Conversion here is done using information from the label: 400,000 U = 250 mg

    $$600,000 \text{ U} \div 400,000 \text{ U/250 mg} = 375 \text{ mg per dose}.$$

    Do the problem:

    $$375 \text{ mg} \div 250 \text{ mg/tablet} = \textbf{1.5 tablets/dose.}$$

9. First, convert:

    $$0.1 \text{ mg} \times 1000 \text{ mcg/mg} = 100 \text{ mcg/dose ordered}.$$

    Do the problem:

    $$100 \text{ mcg} \div 50 \text{ mcg/tablet} = \textbf{2 tablets.}$$

10. First, convert:

$$\text{gr v} = 5 \text{ grains, so gr v} \times 60 \text{ mg/gr} = 300 \text{ mg.}$$

   Do the problem:

$$300 \text{ mg} \div 300 \text{ mg/tablet} = \textbf{1 tablet per dose dispensed.}$$

11. First, convert:

$$\text{gr i ss} = 1.5 \text{ grains, so } 1.5 \text{ grains} \times 60 \text{ mg/grain} = 90 \text{ mg.}$$

   Do the problem:

$$90 \text{ mg/dose} \div 30 \text{ mg/tablet} = \textbf{3 tablets per dose dispensed.}$$

12. No conversion necessary:

$$20 \text{ mEq} \div 10 \text{ mEq/tablet} = \textbf{2 tablets per dose.}$$

13. gr 1/4 = 1/4 grain. 1/4 grain × 60 mg/grain = 15 mg/dose.

   Do the problem:

$$15 \text{ mg/dose} \div 30 \text{ mg/tablet} = \textbf{1/2 tablet.}$$

   Since the tablet is scored in fourths, the dose can be dispensed.

14. gr iss = 1 1/2 grains. Convert grains to mg:

$$1\ 1/2 \text{ grains} \times 60 \text{ mg/grain} = \textbf{90 mg/dose.}$$

   The question asks how many doses are in a bottle containing 500 mg.

$$500 \text{ mg} \div 90 \text{ mg/dose} = \textbf{5 doses.}$$

   (Leftovers do not count.)

15. This is a trick question! Motrin is dispensed as an enteric coated tablet, which cannot be accurately broken. The order cannot be filled.

Chapter 15

Conversion of Liquid Dosage Forms

Quick Study

(See text for full explanation.)

I. **Converting units between dosage *forms* (e.g., solid to liquid dosages)**

   A. *Simplifying the stock concentration*:

   - A stock solution expressed in mg/ml is easier to work with

   C. *Use of fractions*—multiplication and division of fractions

   D. *Using the ratio/proportion method* to convert between liquid and solid dosage forms

   E. *Use of the "order over stock" method*

II. **Converting between percentage solutions and concentrations expressed by ratio**

Converting Between Liquid and Solid Dosage Forms

In the hospital pharmacy, it may be necessary to convert an order for a drug which is expressed in solid amounts (e.g., grams, grains) to a liquid for injection or oral use. For instance, a physician may order furosemide 80 mg po but may ask for the dosage form to be a suspension instead of a tablet. Instead of counting out one 80 mg tablet, you would have to determine the proper amount of suspension to dispense. This is the same type of calculation used to determine the amount of drug to be dispensed for injection as well (see Chapter 16), the difference being that the drug solution or suspension is handled differently.

The type of calculation used for these problems requires a thorough knowledge of fractions, so you may wish to review Chapter 10. Otherwise, the calculations are similar to those covered in Chapter 14, although the ratio/proportion method may be easier to use, for this type of calculation (see below).

Problem: You have an order for 500 mg of cephalexin in suspension. In stock is Keflex suspension, reconstituted to 125 mg/ml. How much would you dispense?

Solution: To do the problem by the "order over stock" method, you need to remember fractions (Chapter 11), especially if the drug concentration is expressed as an amount of drug in a volume of solution that is greater (or less) than 1 ml—for example 2 mg/5 ml:

$$\frac{\text{Order:}\quad 500\ \cancel{mg}}{\text{Stock:}\quad 125\ \cancel{mg}/ml} = 500\ \cancel{mg} \times 1\ ml/125\ \cancel{mg}$$

$$= (500 \times 1\ ml) \div 125\ = 4\ ml$$

Hint: Before working with any problem, if you simplify the stock to get mg/ml, it is easier. If your concentration is in mg/ml, the calculation can be done just like those in Chapter 14—just make the unit mg/ml instead of mg. If conversion is necessary, it is also helpful to simplify the drug concentration before working the problem. (In general, it is a good idea to simplify as much as possible before starting; it saves a lot of time, effort, and potential mistakes.) Let's do a problem that requires conversion.

Problem: You need 50 mg of drug. Your stock is a 5% solution.

Solution:

Step 1:   Convert the units of measurement so that order and stock match. Calculate the concentration of the stock in mg/ml:

5% is 5 g/100 ml (Chapter 12).

The order is in milligrams, so we must convert the 5 g to mg:

5 g = 500 mg, so the concentration of the stock is 5000 mg/100 ml.

Now, simplify: Cancel two zeros on both the top and bottom. The stock concentration is now:

50$\cancel{00}$ mg/1$\cancel{00}$ ml = 50 mg/ml.

Step 2:   Do the calculation.

Order = 50 mg, stock = 50 mg/ml.

Order ÷ stock = 50 mg ÷ (50 mg/ml) = 1 ml to be dispensed.

Now, let's try a problem where the concentration is not so easily simplified.

Problem: You have an order for potassium chloride, 30 mEq po qd. Your stock is KCl 20 mEq/15 ml. Dispense one dose.

Solution: First, simplify as much as possible. The stock concentration can be simplified by dividing both numbers by 5: 20 mEq ÷ 5 = 4 mEq, and 15 ml ÷ 5 = 3 ml, so the stock concentration becomes 4 mEq/3 ml.

Now, we can do the problem. This can be done in one of two ways: the "order over stock" method, or ratio/proportion. Both will be demonstrated.

Dividing the Order by the Stock Concentration

$$\text{Order: } \frac{30 \text{ mEq}}{4 \text{ mEq}/3 \text{ ml}} = 30 \text{ mEq} \times \frac{3 \text{ ml}}{4 \text{ mEq}} = 22.5 \text{ ml}$$

Using Ratio/Proportion

Here we set the two ratios equal to each other and solve algebraically:

$$3 \text{ ml} = 4 \text{ mEq (stock)}$$

$$30 \text{ mEq} = ? \text{ mEq (order)}$$

$$[\text{Order}] \frac{30 \text{ mEq}}{X} = [\text{Stock}] \frac{4 \text{ mEq}}{3 \text{ mL}}$$

The X is going to give us the number of milliliters to dispense. We want to get it by itself on one side of the equation, with numbers on the other side, so we can figure out what it is. So, we first cross-multiply both sides of the equation, and get:

$$30 \text{ mEq} \times 3 \text{ ml} = 4 \text{ mEq} \times \text{dose.}$$

Next, we divide both sides of the equation by 4 mEq, so that we can get the dose by itself on one side:

$$\frac{30 \text{ mEq} \times 3 \text{ ml}}{4 \text{ mEq}} = \text{dose} = 22.5 \text{ ml}$$

Notice that the mEq units cancel out, leaving ml. It is very important that the units which you don't want (mEq, in this case) cancel out in the problem, leaving the units that you do want (ml). *Hint*: Even if you are really not sure how to set up a calculation, if you set it up so that the units you don't want cancel and the ones you do want stay in the problem, it will probably be right. **Units are very important.** If you do not put in and cancel the units, you will have no idea if your calculation is correct!

Notice also that, at the beginning of the ratio/proportion calculation, the two ratios were arranged so that the units on the top of the ratio are the same on both sides of the equal sign, and the units on the bottom of the ratio are also the same on both sides of the equal sign. It does not matter where the units are placed (i.e., on the top or the bottom of the ratio), as long as the placement is the same on both sides, as shown below. For example, the ratio in the problem on the previous page is written correctly, with the units on the top and bottom matching across:

$$\frac{30 \text{ mEq}}{X \text{ ml}} = \frac{4 \text{ mEq}}{3 \text{ ml}}$$

Writing the ratio as:

$$\frac{X \text{ ml}}{30 \text{ mEq}} = \frac{3 \text{ ml}}{4 \text{ mEq}}$$

would also be correct, since units match across the equal sign.
However, writing the ratio as:

$$\frac{30 \text{ mEq}}{X \text{ ml}} = \frac{3 \text{ ml}}{4 \text{ mEq}}$$

would not be correct.

If the ratio is set up properly, the units will cancel, when you cross-multiply. If the units do not cancel properly, the ratios have been set up wrong and need to be corrected.

Problems for Practice

Practice solving the problems by both methods discussed.

1. Your order is for promethazine syrup 12.5 mg po tid. You have a solution in stock which is 6.25 mg/5 ml. What amount is dispensed?

2. Your order is for erythromycin suspension 0.75 g po qid. You have a solution in stock which is 250 mg/5 ml. What amount is dispensed?

3. Your order is for digoxin elixir 0.25 mg qid. You have a solution in stock which is 0.5 mg/10 ml. What amount is dispensed?

4. Your order is for sulfisoxazole susp. 300 mg po stat. You have a solution in stock which is 250 mg/5 ml. What amount is dispensed?

5. Your order is for KCl 20 mEq. You have a solution in stock which is 20 mEq/15 ml. What amount is dispensed?

6. Your order is for cyclosporine 150 mg po. You have a solution in stock which is 100 mg/ml. What amount is dispensed?

7. Your order is for hydrocortizone cypionate susp. 30 mg. You have a solution in stock which is 10 mg/5 ml. What amount is dispensed?

8. Your order is for theophylline 40 mg. You have a solution in stock which is 80 mg/15 ml. What amount is dispensed?

9. Your order is for ampicillin 0.5 g. You have a solution in stock which is 250 mg/2 ml. What amount is dispensed?

10. Your order is for Prozac 10 mg. You have a solution in stock which is 20 mg/5 ml. What amount is dispensed?

11. Your order is for Ceclor 0.25 g. You have a suspension in stock which is 187 mg/5 ml. What amount is dispensed?

12. Your order is for theophylline 120 mg. You have a solution in stock which is 80 mg/5 ml. What amount is dispensed?

13. Your order is for Lasix 40 mg. You have a solution in stock which is 10 mg/ml. What amount is dispensed?

14. Your order is for Polymox 500 mg. You have a solution in stock which is 250 mg/5 ml. What amount is dispensed?

Solutions to Problems for Practice

Many of the problems are calculated in the same way, so only some of the problems will be calculated out. These problems may be done in two ways; dividing the order by the stock available, or using ratio/proportion. Both will be demonstrated.

1. Since the problem does not specify the calculation for a unit dose, the calculation is asking you to determine the amount dispensed for *one* dose. We can calculate this by using either of two ways:

    Order/Stock method: Both order and stock are expressed in the same units (mg), so no conversion is necessary.

    12.5 mg ÷ 6.25 mg/5 ml = 12.5 mg × ml/6.25 mg = 10 ml dispensed (see Chapter 10 for fraction division).

    Ratio/Proportion method

    1. Set up the problem: $\dfrac{12.5 \text{ mg}}{X} = \dfrac{6.25 \text{ mg}}{5 \text{ ml}}$

    2. Cross-multiply: 12.5 mg × 5 ml = 6.25 mg × X

    3. Divide by 6.25 mg to get X.

    Answer: **10 ml**

2. First, *convert* the order into milligrams, to match the stock.

    $$0.75 \text{ g} \times 1000 \text{ mg/g} = 750 \text{ mg for the order.}$$

    Next, *simplify* the stock. This will make the calculation easier:

    $$250 \text{ mg/5 ml} = 50 \text{ mg/ml.}$$

    Now *calculate.* 750 mg ÷ 50 mg/ml = 15 ml dispensed.

    Ratio/proportion: 750 mg/X = 250 mg/5 ml

    $$750 \text{ mg} \times 5 \text{ ml} = 250 \text{ mg} \times X.$$

    Divide both sides by 250 mg:

    $$\frac{750 \text{ mg} \times 5 \text{ ml}}{250 \text{ mg}} = \textbf{15 ml} \text{ dispensed}$$

3. **5 ml** (see Problem 1).

4. **6 ml** (see Problem 1).

5. For this problem, it is important to realize that mEq is just another unit, like mg or ml. Do not let the different unit throw you (it is the same with international units in the next chapter). The problem is done just as Problem 1. Answer: **15 ml.**

6. **1.5 ml** (see Problem 1).

7. **15 ml** (see Problem 1).

8. **7.5 ml** (see Problem 1).

9. First, convert. The order is in grams, the stock in milligrams.

$$0.5 \text{ g} \times 1000 \text{ mg/g} = 500 \text{ mg ordered.}$$

Then, simplify.

$$250 \text{ mg/2 ml} = 125 \text{ mg/ml.}$$

Now, calculate:

$$500 \text{ mg} \div 125 \text{ mg/ml} = \textbf{4 ml.}$$

10. **2.5 ml** (see Problem #1).

11. First, convert. The order is in grams, the stock in milligrams.

$$0.25 \text{ g} \times 1000 \text{ mg/g} = 250 \text{ mg ordered.}$$

This is a weird concentration of stock, which does not simplify. So, we will do this one by ratio/proportion:

$$\frac{250 \text{ mg}}{X} = \frac{187 \text{ mg}}{5 \text{ ml}}$$

Cross-multiply:

$$250 \text{ mg} \times 5 \text{ ml} = 187 \text{ mg} \times X$$

Then divide both sides by 187 mg to get X:

Answer: **6.68 ml**.

12. **7.5 ml** (see Problem 1).

13. **4 ml** (see Problem 1).

14. **10 ml** (see Problem 1).

Chapter 16

Pediatric Doses

Quick Study

(See text for full explanation.)

I. **Computation by body weight in pounds or kilograms**

    A. *(weight of the child × adult dose) ÷ 1.7*

II. **Calculation of dose by body surface area (BSA)**

III. **Young's Rule:**

    A. [age of child in years ÷ (age + 12)] × adult dose

IV. **Clark's Rule:**

    A. [weight of child ÷ (weight of child +150)] × adult dose

V. **The recommended daily dosage range: calculation of safe doses**

    A. Use of the manufacturer's label

Computation of Pediatric Doses—Differences from the Adult Dose

Doses for pediatric patients are calculated differently from adult doses. This is due to the differences in size, weight, and organ development between adults and children. There are several ways to compute a child's dose.

Computation of Dose by Body Weight

The proper dose of drug to administer to a patient (adult or child) can often be calculated as a function of the patient's body weight. The suggested doses for these drugs are often expressed on the manufacturer's label as a number of milligrams per kilogram of body weight. The child's dose will always be smaller than the adult dose, so the adult dose is divided by a conversion factor of 1.7 to obtain the child's dose.

Problem: An adult patient weighs 75 kg. The recommended adult dose is 10 mg/kg. Calculate the dose.

Solution: The weight of the patient is already expressed in kilograms, so no conversion is necessary. Simply multiply the recommended dose in mg/kg by the weight of the patient:

$$75 \text{ kg} \times 10 \text{ mg/kg} = 750 \text{ mg/dose.}$$

It is important not to be confused here by the term *dose*. The adult dose is how much we give the patient per unit of body weight and is used to calculate the patient's actual dose. The patient's dose is how much actual drug is given to the patient, on an individual basis.

Problem: A patient weighs 85 kg. The recommended adult dose for the drug is 2 mg/kg. Calculate the dose for the patient.

Solution: Again, no conversion is necessary. The patient should receive 2 mg for every kg of body weight (85 kg):

$$2 \text{ mg/kg} \times 85 \text{ kg} = 170 \text{ mg/dose.}$$

Calculating a Child's Dose (For Patients Ages 2–12)

Since children should receive only a fraction of the adult dose (due to differences in metabolism, size, etc.), we divide the adult dose by a conversion factor of 1.7, as described previously.

Problem: Using the problem presented above, calculate the dose for a 34 kg child.

Solution: Begin by calculating the adult dose as before:

$$2 \text{ mg/kg} \times 34 \text{ kg} = 68 \text{ mg/dose.}$$

Then divide by the conversion factor to determine the child's dose:

$$68 \text{ mg} \div 1.7 = 40 \text{ mg per child's dose.}$$

Occasionally, we may need to convert the patient's weight (adult or child) into kilograms before beginning the calculation, if it is expressed in pounds.

Problem: A patient weighs 220 lb and receives a drug with a recommended child's dose of 10 mg/kg. Calculate the dose.

Solution: This time, we need to first convert the patient's weight into kilograms. Recall that there are 2.2 lb per kilogram (Chapter 11):

$$220 \text{ lb} \times 2.2 \text{ lb/kg} = 100 \text{ kg.}$$

We use this for the patient's weight and calculate the patient's dose as follows:

$$10 \text{ mg/kg} \times 100 \text{ kg} = 1000 \text{ mg (1 g) of drug per dose.}$$

Computation of Dose by Body Surface Area (BSA)

In this method, the dose is related to the size of the person rather than the weight. The **body surface area (BSA)** is the total area of the surface of the body, as if we were to remove our skin and lay it out to be measured. This way relates the dose to how large the person is. Again, this calculation gives an adult dose, unless it is otherwise specified on the label, and we have to convert to a child's dose, just as we did before.

Body surface area is measured in square meters (m^2). Thus, the recommended dose is given in mg of drug/m^2. We can use the BSA in two ways:

- To check the prescribed dose for safety, divide the dose by the BSA to get mg/m^2. Then compare it to the safe dose range (see below).
- To compute a dose for an individual patient, multiply the dose in mg/m^2 by the BSA (in m^2).

Computation of the BSA

To find the body surface area of a person, we use a **nomogram**. This is a chart that relates the height and weight of a person to his or her body surface area. To use this chart, you will need a ruler. Determine the height and weight of the patient, making sure that the units are in the same system (i.e., height in meters and weight in kilograms, or height in inches with weight in pounds). Find the height of the patient on the scale at the left of the chart, making sure to use the scale in the appropriate units. Then find the weight of the patient on the scale at the right of the chart. Lay the ruler between the two points and draw a line over the top of the ruler. The line will intersect the scale in the middle of the chart. Read the number from this scale, and you have the patient's BSA in m^2. (Since a nomogram is presently not included in the PCTB exam, it will not be presented here. However, any pharmacy math text should have a nomogram for practice. Examinees will, however, be expected to perform calculations relating to body surface area, using information provided.)

Problem: Using a BSA of 0.4 m^2, calculate the dose for a patient prescribed 40 mg/m^2 kanamycin.

Solution: Simply multiply the BSA by the prescribed dose:

$$40 \text{ mg/m}^2 \times 0.4 \text{ m}^2 = 16 \text{ mg.}$$

Problem: The dose calculated above was for an adult. Calculate the child's dose.

Solution: Divide the adult dose by the conversion factor:

$$16 \text{ mg}/1.7 = 9.4 \text{ mg}.$$

Young's Rule and Clark's Rule

There are two other methods for calculating children's doses: Young's Rule and Clark's Rule. *Young's Rule* is easy to remember, because it calculates the dose by the age of the patient (Young–age). *Clark's Rule* relates the dose to the child's weight, as compared to an adult weight of 150 lb.

Young's Rule: $\dfrac{\text{age of child (years)}}{\text{age of child} + 12} \times \text{adult dose} = \text{child's dose}$

Clark's Rule: $\dfrac{\text{weight of child}}{\text{weight} + 150} \times \text{adult dose} = \text{child's dose}$

It would be wise to commit these rules to memory, as they will be on the exam.

Note: Calculations performed by these two methods will not always produce identical answers. Therefore, if you are asked to compute a child's dose by Young's rule and use Clark's rule instead (or another method if you can't remember either one), you will not get the correct answer on the exam.

For example: A child weighs 30 lb and is four years old. Another child is also four years old but weighs 40 lb. The adult dose of Keflex is 250 mg. Calculate both of the children's doses by 1) Young's Rule and 2) Clark's Rule.

Child 1:   Young's Rule: [4 yr/(4 yr + 12)] × 250 mg/dose = 62.5 mg
Clark's Rule: [30 lb/(30 lb + 150)] × 250 mg/dose = 41.7 mg

Child 2:   Young's Rule: produces the same answer as Child 1: 62.5 mg
Clark's Rule: [40 lb/(40 lb+150)] × 250 mg/dose = 52.6 mg

In this case, the results of the two calculations are not the same.

Recommended Daily Doses (Safe Dose)

Occasionally, it may be necessary for the technician to check the dosage prescribed to make sure that it is safe. The *manufacturer's label* carries information about dosage, including the recommended adult dose. This sometimes, but not always, includes the recommended child's dose. It also should include the **safe dose range**. This range of doses gives the amounts that are acceptable for a patient to take. It will look something like "safe dose range: 0.2 mg – 0.8 mg." This means that 0.2 mg, 0.8 mg, or anything in between are acceptable for dosing, but anything below 0.2 mg (which would be ineffective) or above 0.8 mg (which would be toxic) would be unacceptable. The technician may need to perform calculations to check the prescribed dose to be sure that it is safe for the patient to take. (Note: The manufacturer's label may carry, instead of a range, just one "safe dose." Anything at or below this dose is judged to be safe.) If the dose prescribed falls outside of the safe dose range, the problem should be brought to the attention of the pharmacist.

Problem: The dose of amoxicillin prescribed for a 44 lb child is 250 mg qid. The label gives a safe dose range of 15 – 50 mg/kg per day. Is the dose safe?

Solution: First, convert pounds to kilograms: 44 lb ÷ 2.2 lb/kg = 20 kg. Next, divide the 250 mg dose by the child's weight:

$$250 \text{ mg}/20 \text{ kg} = 12.5 \text{ mg/kg}.$$

This is the amount for one dose. The amount prescribed *per day*, however, is four times that amount (qid), or 50 mg. This amount falls within the range of 15–50 mg/kg/day. The dose is safe.

Problem: The recommended child's dose of Keflex is 25 mg/kg/day in two divided doses. If a child weighs 22 lb, how much drug would be prescribed per day?

Solution: First, convert pounds to kilograms: 22 lb ÷ 2.2 lb/kg = 10 kg of body weight. The recommended daily dose for the child is 25 mg/kg/day, so you multiply by the body weight in kg to get the amount of drug actually given:

$$25 \text{ mg/kg} \times 10 \text{ kg} = \textbf{250 mg/day.}$$

Problems for Practice

1. You have an order for kanamycin 40 mg/m^2. A child is 36 inches tall and weighs 30 lb. You calculate the BSA to be 0.6 m^2. Calculate one dose.

2. A child weighing 20 kg is prescribed 10 mg/kg of drug. If this is the adult dose, calculate the proper dose for the child.

3. A child weighs 66 lb. The order is for cloxacillin 250 mg po q6h. The safe dose described on the label is 50 mg/kg/day. Is the dose safe?

4. An adult dose of phenobarbital is 100 mg. Calculate the dose for a child weighing 22 lb.

5. Calculate the dose of phenobarbital for a ten year old child.

6. Your order is for ethambutal 15 mg/kg for a child weighing 22 kg. Calculate one dose.

7. The adult dose for diazepam is 10 mg/m^2. A child is 100 cm tall and weighs 25 kg. You calculate the child's BSA to be 1.25 m^2. Calculate one dose for the child.

8. The child in Problem 7 receives 0.5 mg of Xanax. The safe dosage range is 0.1 – 0.5 mg/m^2. Is the dose safe?

9. An adult dose of Keflin is 1 g. What is the dose for a child weighing 25 lb?

10. Your order is for Narcan neonatal 0.5 mg/kg. The infant weighs 5500 g. Calculate the correct dose for the infant.

11. Your order is for clindamycin 20 mg/kg. The child weighs 88 lb. Your stock is lincomycin 300 mg/ml. How much do you dispense?

12. Your order is for diazepam 0.25 mg/kg. The child weighs 22 lb. Your stock is a 5 mg vial diluted to 2 ml. What amount is dispensed?

13. A child weighs 16 lb, 10 oz. The order is for Lasix 15 mg po bid. The safe dose range is 2–6 mg/kg body weight. Is the dose safe?

14. Adult dose for garamycin is 40 mg/m^2 IM tid. A child is 36 inches tall and weighs 50 lb. You calculate the BSA to be 0.8 m^2. Calculate one dose for the child.

15. A child is eight years old and weighs 50 lb. The adult dose of cephalexin is 250 mg. Use both Clark's Rule and Young's Rule to calculate the child's dose.

Solutions to Problems for Practice

1. The BSA is 0.6 m². Multiply the dose by the BSA to get the dose for the child:
$$40 \text{ mg/m}^2 \times 0.6 \text{ m}^2 = \textbf{24 mg}.$$

2. First multiply weight and prescribed dosage to obtain the *adult* dose:
$$20 \text{ kg} \times 10 \text{ mg/kg} = 200 \text{ mg}.$$

   Next, divide by 1.7, to obtain the proper dose for a child:
$$200 \text{ mg}/1.7 = \textbf{117.6 mg}.$$

3. First, convert pounds to kilograms:
$$\frac{66 \text{ lb}}{2.2 \text{ lb/kg}} = 30 \text{ kg body weight}.$$

   Then, divide body weight and dose:
$$\frac{250 \text{ mg}}{30 \text{ kg}} = \text{dose} = 8.34 \text{ mg/kg}.$$

   Multiply this by four (q6h is four times per day): 8.34 mg/kg × 4 = 33.3 mg/kg. This number falls below the safe dosage guideline on the label (50 mg/kg), so **the dose is safe**.

4. If only the child's weight and the adult dose are given, use Clark's Rule:
$$\frac{22 \text{ lb}}{(22 \text{ lb} + 150)} \times 100 \text{ mg} = \textbf{12.8 mg}.$$

5. If only the child's age and the adult dose are given, use Young's Rule:
$$\frac{10 \text{ years}}{(10 \text{ years} + 12)} \times 100 \text{ mg} = \textbf{45.5 mg}.$$

6. 15 mg/kg × 22 kg = **330 mg**.

7. BSA = 1.25 m², so 10 mg/m² × 1.25 m² = **12.5 mg**.

8. BSA: see Problem 7. Divide 0.5 mg by the BSA = 0.5 mg/1.25 m² = 0.625 mg/m². Now compare this to safe dose range: The dose is above the safe dose range. **It is not safe.**

9. Use Clark's Rule:
$$[25 \text{ lb}/(25 \text{ lb} + 150)] \times 1 \text{ g} = 0.142 \text{ g or } \textbf{142 mg}.$$

10. 5500 g = 5.5 kg. 5.5 kg × 0.5 mg/kg = **2.75 mg**.

11. 88 lb/2.2 lb per kg = 40 kg body weight. 20 mg/kg × 40 kg = 800 mg of drug ordered. Order/stock = 800 mg ÷ 300 mg/ml = **2.67 ml**.

12. 22 lb = 10 kg body weight. 0.25 mg/kg × 10 kg = 2.5 mg/dose ordered. Calculate stock concentration:
$$5 \text{ mg/2 ml} = 2.5 \text{ mg/ml}.$$
$$\text{Order/stock} = 2.5 \text{ mg} \div 2.5 \text{ mg/ml} = \textbf{1.0 ml}.$$

13. 10 oz = 10 oz/16 oz per lb = 0.625 lb. 16.625 lb ÷ 2.2 lb/kg = 7.56 kg body weight. Divide dose by body weight to get mg/kg:

$$15 \text{ mg}/7.56 \text{ kg} = 2 \text{ mg/kg}. \textbf{ The dose is safe}.$$

14. BSA is 0.8 m^2.

$$40 \text{ mg/m}^2 \times 0.8 \text{m}^2 = \textbf{32 mg}.$$

15. Young's Rule:

$$\frac{8 \text{ years}}{(8 \text{ years} + 12)} \times 250 \text{ mg} = \textbf{100 mg}.$$

    Clark's Rule:

$$\frac{50 \text{ lb}}{(50 \text{ lb} + 150)} \times 250 \text{ mg} = \textbf{62.5 mg}.$$

Chapter 17

Parenteral Dosages

Quick Study

(See text for full explanation.)

 I. **Types of parenteral injections and their uses**

 II. **Preparation and use of IV bolus vs. IV drip**

 III. **Drug reconstitution and calculation of drug concentration**

    A. Use of the manufacturer's label

 IV. **Choosing the appropriate syringe and needle for dispensing**

    A. The accuracy of syringe calibrations decreases with increasing size

    B. Use a syringe calibrated to the exact amount to be withdrawn

    C. Choosing the appropriate needle for the type of injection

 V. **Calculation of the correct amount to be dispensed**

    A. Use of percentages and ratios

    B. Preparation of intramuscular and intravenous injections

Parenteral Dosage Forms

There are two ways to administer medication into the body: **enteral**, which means that the medication goes through or into the digestive tract, and **parenteral**, which means that it bypasses the digestive tract and goes into the blood. Parenteral dosage forms refer to anything that is injected; intravenously injected drugs obviously go directly into the blood, but drugs administered by intramuscular and subcutaneous injections do, too, just a little more slowly, which is the purpose of administering them that way. There are several types of parenteral injections. The technician should be familiar with the following types of parenteral injections and their uses:

- Subcutaneous injections (sub-cu, or SC), such as insulin. Drug is injected under the skin.
- Intramuscular injections (IM), such as penicillin.
- Intraarterial injections (IA), these are rare.
- Intrathecal injections (IT). Drug is injected into the space surrounding the spinal cord.
- Intracardiac injections (IC). Drug is injected directly into the heart.
- Intravenous injections (IV). These are the most common, along with IM and sub-cu, and include two forms:
  - the IV bolus (drug is given all at once—one syringe is prepared).
  - the IV drip (given over a long period of time—an IV "bag" or bottle is prepared).

Calculation of Parenteral Doses

Parenteral doses are calculated similarly to the oral doses in Chapter 15; however, these doses are drawn aseptically for injection into the body. Drug concentrations may also be expressed as a percentage or ratio (see Chapter 12), as well as in weight or units per volume. Drug concentration should be given on the manufacturer's label. If it is not, it can be easily calculated. For instance, the label may state that the bottle contains 500 mg of drug, and the volume is 20 ml. A simple division tells us that the concentration of drug in the bottle is 25 mg/ml.

The use of ratio/proportion is helpful in calculations involving liquids for injection.

Problem: The order is for atropine sulfate 0.8 mg, and the available stock is 0.4 mg/ml.

Solution: Set the ratios of the order and stock equal, cross-multiply, and divide, as before:

Step 1. $\dfrac{0.8 \text{ mg}}{X} = \dfrac{0.4 \text{ mg}}{\text{ml}}$

Step 2. $0.8 \text{ mg} \times 1 \text{ ml} = 0.4 \text{ mg} \times X$

Step 3. $(\underset{2}{\cancel{0.8 \text{ mg}}} \times 1 \text{ ml}) \div \underset{1}{\cancel{0.4 \text{ mg}}} = X = \textbf{2 ml}$

Ratio/proportion is especially useful when we have a drug concentration that does not simplify.

Problem: The order is for phenobarbital gr i IM. Available stock is 200 mg/3 ml.

Solution: First, convert: gr i × 60 mg/gr = 60 mg for the order.

Next, calculate:

Step 1. $\dfrac{60 \text{ mg}}{X} = \dfrac{200 \text{ mg}}{3 \text{ ml}}$

Step 2.   60 mg × 3 ml = 200 mg × X

Step 3. $\dfrac{60 \text{ mg} \times 3 \text{ ml}}{200 \text{ mg}} = X$

X = 0.9 ml

Problem: The order is for lidocaine 25 mg subcutaneously. Stock is a 1% solution.

Solution: First, convert the stock:

1% = 1 g/100 ml = 1000 mg/100 ml = 10 mg/ml.

Next, do the problem (we will try the order/stock method):

25 mg ÷ (10 mg/ml) = 2.5 ml.

Syringes

The size of the syringe which is chosen to draw up the medication should be as close as possible to the volume of drug being drawn up, as discussed in Chapter 13. In other words, if you dispense a 1.5 ml dose, choose a 3 ml syringe, not a 5 ml syringe. A 1 ml dose should be dispensed in a 1 ml syringe. The reason for this is that the larger the syringe, the less accurate the markings (see Chapter 13). The accuracy of a syringe is also proportional to its volume, so you should always measure volumes in the closest size of syringe.

Needles

Choosing the proper size of needle is important, too. A large bore needle (16G – 18G) will draw up and dispense quickly so is used for rehydration, dilution, and admixtures. A large bore needle is also necessary to penetrate dense muscle tissue so must be dispensed on a syringe that is to be used for an IM injection. A fine needle (25G–30G) would similarly be needed for subcutaneous injections, to penetrate the more delicate tissues of the skin with a minimum of discomfort, and a medium needle (22G) for IV injections, to penetrate the smooth muscle layer of the vessel without extravasation from the vein.

Using the Manufacturer's Label

The manufacturer's label may contain very useful instructions for dilution and preparation of the drug. For instance, the label on a bottle of penicillin may contain a dilution table which allows you to prepare a specific concentration of drug solution. This allows you to draw up an amount of solution for injection, which contains the proper amount of drug. A sample dilution table follows:

23 ml provides 200,000 Units/ml

18 ml provides 250,000 Units/ml

8 ml provides 500,000 Units/ml

3 ml provides 1,000,000 Units/ml

To use this table, the technician must first decide what volume is needed for the order (an IM injection must be no more than 3 ml in volume, 2 ml is preferable) and compute the concentration needed. Then, that concentration is compared to those listed on the chart, and the proper amount of **diluent** (the water or saline that must be added to the drug to make a solution) is added.

Problem: Using the chart above, prepare an order for 500,000 U penicillin IM.

Solution: We would like to have about 2 ml for an IM injection. The order is for 500,000 U.

500,000 U/2 ml = 250,000 U/ml.

This is the concentration of drug which we want. According to the chart, we can get that concentration by adding 18 ml of water to the vial of drug. We reconstitute with 18 ml of water and draw up 2 ml for the dose.

Problems for Practice

1. Your order is for Demerol 20 mg IM. Available stock is 50 mg/5 ml. Dispense:

2. Your order is for Lanoxin 0.6 mg IV. Available stock is 500 mcg/2 ml. Dispense:

3. Your order is for morphine gr ss. Available stock is 6 mg/ml. Dispense:

4. Your order is for heparin 4000 U SC. Your stock is heparin 10000 U/5 ml. Dispense:

5. Your order is for neostigmine 0.5 mg. Available stock is 1 mg/2 ml. Dispense:

6. Your order is for 50 U of U100 insulin. The pharmacy is out of insulin syringes. How much insulin would you dispense (in ml) using a 1 cc syringe?

7. Your order is for 1 mg of epinephrine. Your stock is a 1:1000 solution. Dispense:

8. Your order is for aminophylline 50 mg. Available stock is 500 mg/20 ml. Dispense:

9. Your order is for Tigan 150 mg. Available stock is 100 mg/ml. Dispense:

10. Your order is for Depo-Provera 0.2 g. Available stock is 500 mg/5 ml vial. Dispense:

11. Your order is for atropine sulfate 0.2 mg. Available stock is 400 mcg/ml. Dispense:

12. Your order is for Vistaril 25 mg. Available stock is 125 mg/5 ml. Dispense:

13. Your order is for 350,000 U of penicillin IM. The manufacturer's label lists a chart of dilutions which is the same as the one on p. 134. How much volume do you add, and how much do you dispense for an IM bolus of 350,000 U?

Solutions to Problems for Practice

1. There are several ways to do this. By the order-over-stock method, first reduce the stock concentration to make the problem simpler: 50 mg/5 ml = 10 mg/ml. Then do the problem:

    $$20 \text{ mg} \div 10 \text{ mg/ml} = \textbf{2 ml.}$$

    By ratio proportion, we simply set the order equal to the stock:

    $$20 \text{ mg}/X = 50 \text{ mg}/5 \text{ ml.}$$

    Cross-multiply and divide: 20 mg × 5 ml/50 mg = **2 ml.**

2. Convert: 0.6 mg × 1000 mcg/mg = 600 mcg. Then do the problem:

    $$600 \text{ mcg} \div 500 \text{ mcg}/2 \text{ ml} = (600 \text{ mcg} \times 2 \text{ ml})/500 \text{ mcg} = \textbf{2.4 ml.}$$

3. gr ss = 1/2 gr. 1/2 grain × 60 mg/gr = 30 mg. 30 mg ÷ 6 mg/ml = **5 ml.**

4. Simplify the stock: 10000 U/5 ml = 2000 U/ml.

    Divide: 4000 U ÷ 2000 U/ml = **2 ml.**

5. This could be done using order-over-stock, but let's try the ratio/proportion method:

    $$0.5 \text{ mg}/X = 1 \text{ mg}/2 \text{ ml.}$$

    Cross-multiply and divide:

    $$\frac{0.5 \text{ mg} \times 2 \text{ ml}}{1 \text{ mg}} = \frac{X \times 1 \text{ mg}}{1 \text{ mg}} = 0.5 \times 2 \text{ ml} = \textbf{1 ml.}$$

6. A 1cc syringe holds 100 U of regular (U100) insulin: 1 ml = 100 U, so, by ratio/proportion, 50 U/100 U = X/1 ml. Dispense **0.5 ml** of insulin.

7. 1:1000 = 1 g/1000 ml = 1 mg/ml (see Chapter 11). Order is for 1 mg. 1 mg ÷ 1 mg/ml = **1 ml.**

8. First, reduce the stock: 500 mg/20 ml = 25 mg/ml. Then divide: 50 mg ÷ 25 mg/ml = **2 ml.**

9. No reduction is necessary: 150 mg ÷ 100 mg/ml = **1.5 ml.**

10. First, convert: 0.2 g × 1000 mg/g = 200 mg.

    Then simplify stock: 300 mg/3 ml = 100 mg/ml.

    Now calculate: 200 mg ÷ 100 mg/ml = **2 ml** dispensed.

11. First, convert: 0.2 mg × 1000 mcg/mg = 200 mcg ordered.

    Calculate: 200 mcg/400 mcg/ml = **0.5 ml** dispensed.

12. 25 mg/X = 125 mg/5 ml.

    Cross-multiply: 25 mg × 5 ml = 125 mg × X

    Divide to get X: (25 mg × 5 ml)/125 mg = X = 1 ml dispensed.

13. You want a volume of around 2 ml (1–3 ml) to inject for an IM injection. Do the order/stock calculation for each concentration given on the label, for example, 350,000 U/1,000,000 U/ml = 0.35 ml, 350,000 U/500,000 U/ml = 0.7 ml. When you reach the concentration that gives around 2 ml for the injection volume, this is the concentration which you want. In this case, the closest volume to be calculated is from the 200,000 U/ml concentration, which we would get by adding 23 ml to the bottle: 350,000 U/200,000 U/ml = **1.75 ml.** The problem with this answer is that we would have to use a 5 ml syringe, which is only calibrated in tenths, and we would have to extrapolate ("guestimate") 1.75 ml. So, we try the 250,000 U/ml concentration: 350,000 U/250,000 U/ml = **1.4 ml** to be injected. Now, simply plan to follow the instructions on the label: add 18 ml of diluent, and then draw up 1.4 ml to fill the order.

Chapter 18

Intravenous calculations

Quick Study

(See text for full explanation.)

I. **Calculation of flow rate**

    A. *Volume* per *Time (V/T) = ml/time*

       • Useful in dose/time calculations

    B. $\dfrac{V}{T} \times drop\ factor = drops\ per\ time$

       • Used for proper choice of infusion set

II. **Types of fluids administered**

    A. Salt solutions

    B. Sugar solutions

    C. Solutions for irrigation

    D. Addition of potassium or drug admixtures

Administering Intravenous Medication—The IV Drip

Intravenous drugs are administered in two ways: the bolus, which is an injection given all at once, and the IV drip, which is administered over a long period of time. We discussed the bolus injections in Chapter 16. We will now discuss the IV drip calculations.

The first thing that we need to be concerned with is the concept of **flow rate**. When a patient is connected to an IV drip, the fluid flows in at a particular rate. The rate of flow is set by a "controller" or mechanical device, or by an **infusion set**, which consists of a plastic barrel connected to plastic tubing. One end of the barrel is inserted into the IV bag, and the other leads into the tubing which connects to the needle inserted in the patient. An infusion set is calibrated to deliver a drop of a certain size (expressed as a number drops *per milliliter*). The rate at which the drops flow into the tubing (and thus the patient) is adjusted manually by the nurse or technician. The size of the drop is determined by the **drop factor** and determines how much of the IV solution goes into the patient per unit of time. Infusion sets come in 10 gtt/ml, 15 gtt/ml, and 60 gtt/ml sizes.

Solutions that are normally infused include:

- Normal saline (NS), which is 0.9% sodium chloride (salt)
- 1/2 normal saline (1/2 NS), which is 0.45% sodium chloride
- 1/4 normal saline (1/4 NS), which is 0.225% sodium chloride
- 5% dextrose (glucose, a sugar) in water (D_5W)
- Any of the above saline solutions with potassium chloride added. These are labeled in red, as potassium overdose can be lethal. Red print labeling is easy to see and helps to prevent accidental potassium overdosage.

Various drugs may be added to these solutions for slow infusion (IV admixtures, see Chapter 19), or a small IV bag (piggyback IV) containing a drug solution may be hung with the IV bag to slowly release drug into the patient's system.

Flow Rate

Flow rate is volume per time. To determine the flow rate, simply take the volume of fluid that is flowing into the patient and divide it by the time that it takes to flow in. These calculations will be very useful in calculating dose and dose per time (Chapters 19 and 20).

Example: A patient receives 250 ml of normal saline in 2 hr. What is the flow rate?

Solution: Volume ÷ time = 250 ml/2 hr = 125 ml/hr. Sometimes the flow rate is needed in minutes. In this case, we must convert hours to minutes before dividing (2 hr ÷ 60 min/hr).

Calculating flow rate in drops per time using an infusion apparatus.

Calculating flow rate by drops requires an extra calculation. We calculate the flow rate in milliliters just as before. However, we are now calculating the number of drops per time, so we need to take the drop factor into account. The drop factor calibration of the infusion set is designated by a number printed on the package. This number allows us to calculate how much volume is contained per drop. The volume infused in milliliters per time divided by the number of drops per milliliter (the drop factor) gives us the flow rate in drops per time. This calculation is necessary to determine which infusion set to include with an IV set and to calculate volume flow rate counting the number of drops that flow through the infusion set per time.

Calculating Drops per Time (Drop Rate)

Remember: (Volume ÷ time) × drop factor = drops per time.

Problem: An order states that 100,000 U of penicillin is to be added to a one liter bag of saline and infused in five hours. Your infusion set is labeled 10 gtt/ml. What is the flow rate in gtt/min?

Solution: 1 L of NS is infused in 5 hours, so flow rate is:

$$1000 \text{ ml}/5 \text{ hr} = 200 \text{ ml}/\text{hr}.$$

We want the rate in minutes, so, since there are 60 min in one hour, this becomes:

$$200 \text{ ml}/60 \text{ min or } 3.33 \text{ ml}/\text{min}.$$

Now, we need to change milliliters to drops:

$$3.33 \text{ ml}/\text{min} \times 10 \text{ gtt}/\text{ml} = 33.3 \text{ gtt}/\text{min}.$$

Since we cannot have a fraction of a drop, this becomes just 33 gtt/min.

If we have the flow rate in drops per time and need to do a calculation, we can easily convert the flow rate back to milliliters per time:

Problem: We have a flow rate of 20 gtt/min. The infusion apparatus is a *macrodrip* (10 gtt/ml). What is the flow rate in ml/hr?

Solution: First, we change drops to milliliters:

$$20 \text{ gtt}/\text{min} \div 10 \text{ gtt}/\text{ml} = 2 \text{ ml}/\text{min}.$$

Note that we *divided* by the drop factor this time; we multiplied to convert milliliters to drops, and we now divide to convert drops to milliliters.

$$2 \text{ ml}/\text{min} \times 60 \text{ min}/\text{hr} = 120 \text{ ml}/\text{hr}.$$

Problems for Practice

1. 1 L of saline is administered over 10 hours. Find the flow rate in (a) ml per hour and (b) ml/min.
2. The infusion set used with the IV bag in Problem 1 states that the drop factor is 15 gtt/ml. Calculate the flow rate in gtt/min.
3. 500 ml of D_5W runs for 4 hours. Calculate the flow rate in ml/hr and ml/min.

4. 1 L of NS runs for 16 hour, 40 min. Calculate the flow rate in ml/hr and ml/min.

5. You have an order for aminophylline 250 mg in 250 ml NS to run for 8 hr. The drop factor is 60 gtt/ml. What is the flow rate in drops per minute?

6. The order is for 150 ml of NS infused over 3 hr. The infusion set says 60 gtt/ml. Calculate the flow rate in gtt/min.

7. 1 L of NS is infused at 100 ml/hr. How long will the infusion go?

8. 300 ml of Lactated Ringer's solution is infused in 5 hr. The flow rate is 15 gtt/min. What is the drop factor?

9. 1 L of saline runs for 10 hr at 1000 gtt/hr. Calculate the drop factor.

10. 600 ml of Ringer's Lactate runs for 10 hr. The flow rate is 60 gtt/min. Calculate the drop factor.

11. You have a bag of saline with an infusion apparatus labeled 15 gtt/ml. The flow rate is 60 gtt/min. What is the hourly rate of infusion (how much saline will flow into the patient in an hour)?

12. You have 1 L saline, which is to be infused in 6 hr. Available are 10 gtt/ml and 15 gtt/ml infusion sets. Calculate the flow rate for each in gtt/min.

13. 1 L of saline is infusing at 100 ml/hr. How much saline does the patient get in 40 min?

14. 120 ml of NS is to be administered in 30 min using an infusion set labeled 15 gtt/ml. What is the flow rate in gtt/min?

15. 300 ml of D_5W 1/2 NS is delivered in 90 min. Your drop factor is 10 gtt/ml. Calculate the flow rate in gtt/min.

Solutions to Problems for Practice

1. (a) 1L = 1000 ml

    1000 ml/10 hr = **100 ml/hr.**

    (b) 100 ml/hr × 1 hr/60 min = **1.67 ml/min.**

2. flow rate in ml/min = 1.67.

    1.67 ml/min × 15 gtt/ml = **25 gtt/min.**

3. 500 ml/4 hr = **125 ml/hr.**

    125 ml/hr × 1 hr/60 min = **2.08 ml/min.**

4. 40 min × 1 hr/60 min = 0.67 hr.

    Running time = 16.67 hr.

    1 L = 1000 ml.

    1000 ml/16.67 hr = **60 ml/hr.**

    60 ml/hr × 1 hr/60min = **1 ml/min.**

5. Ignore the drug as it is not pertinent to the problem; the question merely asks the flow rate of the saline.

    250 ml/8 hr = 31.25 ml/hr.

    31.25 ml/hr × 1 hr/60 min = 0.52 ml/min.

    0.52 ml/min × 60 gtt/ml = **31 gtt/min.**

6. 150 ml/3 hr = 50 ml/hr.

    50 ml/hr × 1 hr/60 min = 0.83 ml/min.

    0.83 ml/min × 60 gtt/ml = **50 gtt/min.**

7. 1 L = 1000 ml.

    1000 ml ÷ 100 ml/hr = **10 hr.**

8. 300 ml/5 hr = 60 ml/hr.

    60 ml/hr × 1 hr/60 min = 1 ml/min.

    We want gtt/ml, so arrange the numbers so that the minutes cancel:

    $$\frac{15 \text{ gtt/min}}{1 \text{ ml/min}} = \textbf{15 gtt/ml.}$$

9. Simply figure the flow rate in ml/hr, then divide by the flow rate in gtt/hr:

    1 L = 1000 ml. 1000 ml/10 hr = 100 ml/hr.

    We want the hours to cancel, to get gtt/ml:

    1000 gtt/hr ÷ 100 ml/hr = **10 gtt/ml.**

10. This is done the same way as Problem 9. Flow rate = 600 ml/10 hr = 60 ml/hr.

    60 ml/hr × 1 hr/60min = 1 ml/min.

    60 gtt/min ÷ 1 ml/min = **60 gtt/ml.**

11. Flow rate (gtt/time)/drop factor = flow rate (ml/time):

    60 g̶tt/min ÷ 15 g̶tt/ml = 4 ml/min.

    The hourly rate is the amount per hour, so:

    4 ml/min × 60 min/hr = **240 ml/hr**.

12. 1 L = 1000 ml, and 6 hr = 360 min.

    Flow rate = 1000 ml/360 min = 2.78 ml/min.

    (a) 10 gtt/ml × 2.78 ml/min = **28 gtt/min**.

    (b) 15 gtt/ml × 2.78 ml/min = **42 gtt/min**.

13. (100 ml/hr) × (1 hr/60 min) × 40 min = **66.67 ml**.

14. First, calculate the flow rate in ml/min. Volume/time = 120 ml/30 min = 40 ml/min. Next, calculate flow rate in gtt/min: 40 m̶l/min × 15 gtt/m̶l = **60 gtt/min.**

15. Similar to Problem 14:

    (300 ml/90 min) × 10 gtt/ml = **33 gtt/min**.

Chapter 19

Intravenous Admixtures

Quick Study

(See text for full explanation.)

I. **Calculation of the amount of fluid to be added for reconstitution of drugs**

 A. Calculation of the proper amount to add to reach a desired concentration

 - *Concentration × volume = amount of drug*

 B. Calculation of the concentration reached upon adding a particular amount of diluent

 - Addition of too much diluent by mistake—backcalculating the concentration

 - Determining the proper amount of diluent to add, based on the volume of drug

II. **Calculating the amount of drug to be added to an IV ("admixture")**

 A. *Drugs ordered in units, mg, etc.*

 B. *Drugs ordered in percent*—converting percentage solutions

 - Making a percentage solution from a stock solution using an IV bag

 - Adding the appropriate amount of drug to an IV bag using a percentage solution as stock

Infusing Medications Over Time—The IV Drip and Admixture

Occasionally, it may be necessary for the patient to receive a drug or medication slowly, over a period of hours. In this case, the technician may be asked to prepare an IV solution that contains the proper dosage of drug to be delivered over time. For example, the order might read "Penicillin G K 100,000 U in 1 L NS," or "Heparin Sulfate 1000 U/hr in D_5W." The amount of drug to be added must be calculated and the drugs appropriately rehydrated and added to the IV.

Rehydration and Reconstitution of Drugs

Many drugs are unstable if mixed with water. These drugs are supplied in powder form and must be rehydrated before use. Drugs are always supplied in a salt solution that is **isotonic** to the body; in other words, the concentration of salt in the solution is the same as in the body fluids so that introducing the drug solution into the body will neither dehydrate nor overhydrate the cells. If the drug is already mixed with the salts necessary to make the solution, the technician need only add water to the dry powder. This is called **rehydration**, as we are only giving back the water to the original solution. If the vial contains only the drug or the drug with some extra ingredients to help it work, the instructions may be to add another **diluent** (something that we dilute with) to the powder, such as saline, distilled water, or another salt solution. This is called **reconstitution**. Once diluted, the drug has a limited shelf life, which may be extended by refrigeration.

Problem: The label on a drug vial says to reconstitute with 8 ml of water to get 10 ml of a 500,000 U/ml solution. You add 10 ml to the vial by mistake. What would be the resulting concentration of drug?

Solution: If you had added the correct amount, the label says that you would have had 10 ml of a 500,000 U/ml solution. That being the case, there are:

$$10 \text{ ml} \times 500,000 \text{ U/ml} = 5,000,000 \text{ U in the whole vial}$$
$$(\text{concentration} \times \text{volume} = \text{amount of drug})$$

Now, all we have to do is recalculate, using the new dilution; we are now adding 10 ml instead of 8, so the total volume is now 12 ml instead of 10 (the extra 2 ml is the volume that the drug takes up, which does not change). Now calculate the concentration:

$$5,000,000 \text{ U/vial} \div 12 \text{ ml} = \textbf{416,667 U/ml.}$$

Problem: The order is for penicillin G K 500,000 U to be delivered over 10 hr. A vial of penicillin contains 10,000,000 U in dry form, which must be rehydrated. You have 1 L bags of saline available. Calculate the amount of penicillin to add to the IV.

Solution: We want to add as small a volume as possible to the bag, so as not to change its volume. About 1 to 5 ml would be about right. Let us set up a ratio proportion to calculate the amount to add to the penicillin vial so that we may withdraw 1 ml that contains 500,000 U of drug:

$$\frac{500,000 \text{ U}}{1 \text{ ml}} = \frac{10,000,000 \text{ U}}{X \text{ ml}}$$

Cross multiply and divide:

$$500,000 \times X \text{ ml} = 1 \text{ ml} \times 10,000,000 \text{ U} = 20 \text{ ml}.$$

We add 20 ml to the vial and withdraw 1 ml for injection into the IV bag.

Occasionally, the technician may be asked to add an appropriate amount of drug to an IV bag which results in a particular concentration. In this case, use ratio proportion to determine how much of a particular drug or drug solution is to be added.

Problem: The order is for 250 ml of a 2% calcium gluconate solution in 1/2 NS to be delivered in 5 hours. You have a 20% solution of calcium gluconate on hand. How much do you add to the IV bag?

Solution: First, calculate the amount needed in grams:

$$2\% = 2 \text{ g}/100 \text{ ml}$$

Set up ratio/proportion:

$$\frac{2 \text{ g}}{100 \text{ ml}} = \frac{X \text{ g}}{250 \text{ ml}}$$

Cross multiply and divide:

$$\frac{2 \text{g} \times 250 \text{ ml} = 100 \text{ ml} \times X}{100 \text{ ml}} \quad 5 \text{ g is needed.}$$

Now, determine how much of the 20% solution should be added to the bag:

$$\frac{20 \text{g}}{100 \text{ ml}} = \frac{5 \text{g}}{X}$$

$$X = \frac{500 \text{ g/ml}}{20 \text{ g}} = 25 \text{ ml of the 20% solution is added}$$

Problem: The order is for heparin, 1000 U/hr in 1 L D_5W, to be infused for 5 hours. Calculate the amount of heparin to add to the IV.

Solution: The order states that the dose is 1000 U/hr for 5 hr. The amount to be added is therefore:

$$1000 \text{ U/hr} \times 5 \text{ hr} = 5000 \text{ U}.$$

Problems for Practice

1. The order is for aminophylline 250 mg in 500 ml NS, to run for 8 hr. You have aminophylline 500 mg/5 ml on hand. How much do you put in the IV bag?

2. What is the final concentration of drug in the IV bag prepared in Problem 1?

3. You add 10 ml of 10% calcium gluconate to a 1 L bag of D_5W. What is the concentration of calcium gluconate in the bag?

4. How much dextrose is contained in 300 ml of D_5W?

5. How many milliequivalents of sodium are in 100 ml of saline? Molecular weight of sodium = 23, chlorine = 35.

6. How many milligrams of drug are in 10 ml of a 1:1000 solution?

7. A drug label states that the addition of 8 ml of saline to the vial will result in a drug concentration of 250 mg/ml. You realize that you just added 13 ml to the vial. What is the concentration?

8. You reconstitute a vial of drug with 2.5 ml of saline. The vial contains 2,500,000 U of drug. What is the final concentration of drug in the vial?

9. Your vial of potassium solution contains 20 mEq of potassium per 5 ml. You add 5 ml to a 1 L IV bag. What is the final concentration of potassium in the bag?

10. You reconstitute 1,000,000 U of penicillin with 20 ml of saline. What is the final concentration?

11. What is the concentration of a 1% solution of potassium chloride, in mEq/ml? Molecular weights: potassium = 39 g, chloride = 35.45 g.

12. You add 5 ml of a 250 mg/ml solution of methotrexate to 250 ml of saline. What is the final concentration of drug in the bag?

Solutions to Problems for Practice

1. This is a trick question. The problem states how much to put in the bag: 250 mg. No calculation is necessary. To do order/stock, first reduce the stock:

    $$500 \text{ mg}/5 \text{ ml} = 100 \text{ mg/ml}.$$

    Then, do order over stock:

    $$250 \text{ mg}/100 \text{ mg/ml} = \textbf{2.5 ml}$$

2. Concentration is always amount per volume: amount = 250 mg, volume = 500 ml

    $$C = 250 \text{ mg}/500 \text{ ml} = \textbf{0.5 mg/ml.}$$

3. First, figure how much drug is added:

    $$10 \text{ ml} \times 10 \text{ g}/100 \text{ ml} = 1 \text{ g of drug.}$$

    Next, figure concentration:

    $$1 \text{ g} = 1000 \text{ mg and } 1 \text{ L} = 1000 \text{ ml, so } 1000 \text{ mg}/1000 \text{ ml} = \textbf{1 mg/ml.}$$

4. For this, you must know that D_5W is 5% dextrose:

    $$5 \text{ g}/100 \text{ ml} \times 300 \text{ ml} = \textbf{15 g.}$$

5. Recall that normal saline is 0.9% sodium chloride, and that 0.9% is 0.9 g/100 ml. To determine equivalent weight (Eq, or equivalents), add the molecular weights: 23 g for sodium + 35 g for chloride (chlorine) = 58 g. This is equal to one equivalent. One *milli*equivalent (mEq) would be 1/1000 of that, or 58 mg. 0.9 g = 900 mg, so to determine the number of mEq in 100 ml, we divide the 900 mg by 58 mg/mEq. There are **15.5 mEq** of sodium in 100 ml of saline.

6. 1:1000 is 1 g/1000 ml = 1000 mg/1000 ml = 1 mg/ml (you should memorize this!) so 10 ml × 1 mg/ml = **10 mg.**

7. Because a greater amount of saline was added to the vial, the final concentration will be less. So, we set up the problem:

    $$\frac{8 \text{ ml}}{13 \text{ ml}} \times \frac{250 \text{ mg}}{\text{ml}} = \textbf{153 mg/ml.}$$

8. 2,500,000 U/2.5 ml = **1,000,000 U/ml.**

9. First, determine how much is added:

    $$20 \text{ mEq}/5 \text{ ml} = 4 \text{ mEq/ml.}$$

    You use 5 ml, so 5 ml × 4 mEq/ml = 20 mEq added to the 1 L bag.

    $$\frac{\overset{1}{\cancel{20} \text{ mEq}}}{\underset{50}{\cancel{1000} \text{ ml}}} = \textbf{0.02 mEq/ml.}$$

10. 1,000,000 U/20 ml = 50000 U/ml.

11. Again, convert percentage into mg/ml: 1% = 1g/100 ml = 1000 mg/100 ml = 10 mg/ml.

    So in 10 ml, there are 100 mg.

    1 Eq of KCl = 39 g + 35 g = 74 g, so 1 mEq = 74 mg.

    To determine the number of mEq of potassium present in 10 ml, we simply divide:

    $$\frac{100 \text{ mg}}{74 \text{ mg}} = \textbf{1.34 mEq.}$$

12. 5 ml × 250 mg/ml = 1250 mg of drug added to 250 ml saline. Concentration = 1250 mg/250 ml = **5 mg/ml.**

Calculation of Dose per Time

Calculating the Amount of Drug Infused per Time (Dose per Time)

Calculation of the amount of drug received per time, or dose per time, is simply a matter of using the following formula, which you should memorize:

$$\text{Concentration} \times \text{Flow rate} = \text{Dose/time}$$
$$(C \times F = D/t)$$

The amount of drug per volume of fluid (C), multiplied by how fast the fluid flows into the patient, indicates the amount of drug flowing into the patient per time. When doing these calculations, remember that **dose** refers to the amount of **drug**, not the volume of fluid. Thus, your answer will always come out in a **weight** measurement (e.g., g/hr, mg/min, etc.). This formula is very versatile, and can be used to calculate any of the parameters (C, F, or D/t), as shown below.

Problem: You have a one liter bag of saline containing 1.5 g of antibiotic. The flow rate is 100 ml/hr. What is the hourly dose?

Solution: First, calculate the concentration (amount of drug per volume). Convert: 1.5 g = 1500 mg. The volume of the bag is one liter (1000 ml), so the concentration is 1500 mg/1000 ml = 1.5 mg/ml.

Next, determine the flow rate. It is given in the problem: 100 ml/hr. Finally, multiply:

$$C \times F = D/t = 1.5 \text{ mg/ml} \times 100 \text{ ml/hr} = 150 \text{ mg/hr.}$$

Problem: You have 500 ml D_5W containing 10000 U of heparin. The order states that the patient is to receive 2000 U of heparin per hour. Calculate the flow rate needed (in ml/hr).

Solution: Again, use the formula. The dose per time is given and you can calculate the concentration. Using the formula, solve for the flow rate:

Concentration: drug per volume = 10000 U/500 ml = 20 U/ml.

$C \times F = D/t$:

$$20 \text{ U/ml} \times F = 2000 \text{ U/hr}$$

$$F = \frac{2000 \text{ U/hr}}{20 \text{ U/ml}} = 100 \text{ ml/hr}$$

Problem: A 1L bag of 1/2 NS contains 1000 mEq of potassium. The flow rate is 25 gtt/min, and the drop factor is 15 gtt/ml. What is the hourly dose of potassium?

Solution: Use $C \times F = D/t$.

First, calculate the flow rate in ml/hr:

$$25 \text{ gtt/min} \div 15 \text{ gtt/ml} =$$
$$1.776 \text{ ml/min} \times 60 \text{ min/hr} = 100 \text{ ml/hr}$$

Next, calculate the concentration:

$$1000 \text{ mEq/1000 ml} = 1 \text{ mEq/ml.}$$

Multiply the concentration by the flow rate:

$$1 \text{ mEq/ml} \times 100 \text{ ml/hr} = 100 \text{ mEq/hr.}$$

Problem: A 0.5% solution of lidocaine is flowing at 50 ml per hour. What is the hourly dose?

Solution: There is an easy shortcut to this problem.

First, convert: 0.5% = 0.5 g/100 ml.

Next, use ratio/proportion (or just think and divide):

$$0.5 \text{ g/100 ml} = X \text{ g/50 ml.}$$

Since 50 ml goes into the patient per hour, the hourly dose is obtained by cross-multiplying the above equation and solving for X:

$$X = (0.5 \text{ g/100 ml}) \times 50 \text{ ml} = 0.25 \text{ g or } 250 \text{ mg/hr.}$$

Problems for Practice

1. You have an order for aminophylline, 500 mg in 250 ml D$_5$W, to run for 5 hr. The drop factor is 60 gtt/ml.
   (a) What is the flow rate in gtt/min?
   (b) What is the dose per minute?

2. An IV solution of heparin contains 5000 U in 500 ml and takes 2 hr to infuse. How much drug is infused in 30 min?

3. The solution in Problem 2 (5000 U/500 ml) is to be infused so that the patient gets 1000 U of heparin per hour. Calculate the flow rate in ml/hr.

4. You add 10 ml of a 10% solution of calcium gluconate to a 500 ml IV bag. The flow rate is 30 gtt/min with an infusion set labeled 15 gtt/ml. How much drug does the patient get per hour?

5. An IV solution of a 1% potassium chloride solution infuses at 50 ml/hr. In two hours, how many mEq of potassium does the patient get?

6. A solution of 10000 U of heparin in 500 ml of D$_5$W infuses in eight hours. What is the hourly dose?

7. You add 5 g of drug to 1 L of saline. The hourly dose is to be 250 mg. Calculate the flow rate. How long will the IV run?

8. You add 1 g of aminophylline to 1 L of NS. The patient is to receive 50 mg/hr. What is the flow rate?

9. You have a solution of 0.5% calcium gluconate, which infuses at 100 ml/hr. Calculate the hourly dose.

Solutions to Problems for Practice

1. The infusion is 250 ml to run for 5 hr, so the flow rate is:

   250 ml/5 hr = 50 ml/hr = 0.833 ml/min.

   Flow rate × drop factor = gtt/time, so 0.833 ml/min × 60 gtt/ml = **50 gtt/min**.

   Dose per minute = 0.833 ml/min × (500 mg/250 ml) = **1.67 mg/min**.

2. The long way to approach this problem:

   C = 5000 U/500 ml = 10 U/ml,

   F = 500 ml/2 hr = 250 ml/hr

   D/t = 10 U/ml × 250 ml/hr = 2500 U/hr, or **1250 U in 30 min.**

   Shortcut: 5000 U infuse in two hours, so 2500 U infuse per hour. Therefore, 1250 U would infuse in half an hour (30 min).

3. C = 10 U/ml and D/t = 1000 U/hr, so:

   F = 1000 U/hr ÷ 10 U/ml = **100 ml/hr.**

4. Amount of drug added to the bag:

   10 ml × 10 g/100 ml = 1 g of drug into 500 ml. The concentration is 1000 mg/500 ml = 2 mg/ml.

   The flow rate is 30 gtt/min ÷ 15 gtt/ml = 2 ml/min.

   2 ml/min × 60 min/hr = 120 ml/hr.

   Dose per hour is therefore 2 mg/ml × 120 ml/hr = **240 mg/hr.**

5. 1% = 1 g/100 ml. Since 50 ml/hr infuses, the dose is 0.5 g/hr, or 500 mg. In 2 hr, the patient would get 1000 mg. 1 Eq of potassium (chloride) is 39 g + 35.45 g = 74.45 g, so one milliequivalent would be 74.45 mg. The patient gets 1000 mg, so to convert to mEq, we must divide: 1000 mg/74.45 mg per mEq = **13.4 mEq.**

6. 10000 U/8 hr = **1,250 U/hr.**

7. 5 g = 5000 mg, so C = 5000 mg/1000 ml = 5 mg/ml. Dose/hr = 250 mg/hr, so using **C × F = D/t**, F = 5 mg/ml × F = 250 mg/hr = **50 ml/hr.**

   At 50 ml/hr, the 1000 ml IV will run:

   $$1000 \text{ ml} \div 50 \text{ ml/hr} = \textbf{20 hr.}$$

8. C = 1000 mg/1000 ml = 1 mg/ml. D/t = 50 mg/hr, so using **C × F = D/t**:

   $$F = 50 \text{ mg/hr} \div 1 \text{ mg/ml} = \textbf{50 ml/hr.}$$

9. C = 0.5% = 500 mg/100 ml = 5 mg/ml. F = 100 ml/hr, so using **C × F = D/t**, the hourly dose = 5 mg/ml × 100 ml/hr = **500 mg/hr.**

Chapter 21

Bulk Compounding

Quick Study

(See text for full explanation.)

I. **Types of compounding**

    A. *Bulk compounding*—the compiling of drug product *for general use,* according to a specific, written procedure. This may be legally performed by the technician

    B. *Extemporaneous compounding*—the compiling of a drug product *for a specific patient,* where no written procedure exists. This may only be *done by the pharmacist.*

II. **Reducing and enlarging formulas**

    A. Use of a conversion factor to change amounts of individual ingredients in a formula

    B. Calculating conversion factors: *amount needed ÷ amount specified in the procedure*

III. **Preparing drug products using formulae based on weight and by percentage**

Compounding Drugs by Procedure

On occasion, it may be necessary to make a drug formulation "from scratch." It is permissible for the technician to do this, if a written procedure exists for making the product. This is called **bulk compounding**.

If no procedure exists for making the formulation, the drug product must then be made by the *pharmacist.* Perhaps a physician wants a drug which is normally given orally to be put into suppository form for a patient who is NPO (receives nothing by mouth) or a drug for oral dosage is made into a cream. This type of compounding requires the professional judgment of the pharmacist, and is called *extemporaneous compounding,* where a special drug dosage form is made *for a particular patient.*

When compounding a drug formulation, it is sometimes necessary to reduce or enlarge the formula, according to the amount of drug needed. Let's start with a problem which requires enlarging the formula.

Example: A procedure for making 500 g of antibiotic ointment is as follows:

Neomycin	2.5 g
Bacitracin	4.0 g
Polymixin B	320 mg
Liquid petrolatum	150 g
White petrolatum	343.18 g

In our pharmacy, the antibiotic ointment is a big seller, and 500 g is not enough. We need to make 1000 g. To find out how much of each component to add in order to make 1000 g of ointment instead of 500 g, we must multiply the amount of each ingredient listed in the procedure by a **conversion factor,** a number that will allow the ingredients, when mixed together, to equal 1000 g of ointment.

We determine this conversion factor by *dividing the amount needed by the amount specified in the procedure.* In this case, combining the specified amounts of each ingredient in the procedure will give us 500 g of ointment, and we need 1000 g: 1000 g/500 g = 2. So, we multiply the amounts of all of the ingredients by 2. The enlarged "recipe" for 1000 g of ointment looks like this:

Neomycin	5 g
Bacitracin	8.0 g
Polymixin B	640 mg
Liquid petrolatum	300 g
White petrolatum	686.36 g

Now, suppose that the antibiotic cream doesn't sell well. We now want to make less than the procedure specifies. We only want to make 200 g from the procedure that makes 500 g.

Step 1: Calculate the conversion factor. The amount needed = 200 g. The amount specified in the procedure = 500 g: 200 g/500 g = 0.4. We now multiply all of the original amounts by 0.4, to obtain:

Neomycin	1 g
Bacitracin	1.6 g
Polymixin B	128 mg
Liquid petrolatum	60 g
White petrolatum	137.2 g
To make 200 g	

Making Preparations by Percentage

A procedure for preparing a drug formulation may be expressed in percentages. If this is the case, you will have to convert the percentages to numerical form first, before measuring or calculating.

Example: A procedure for preparing calamine lotion reads as follows:

Calamine	8%
Zinc oxide	8%
Glycerol	2%
Bentonite	25%

q.s. (fill to the proper volume) with 2% calcium hydroxide solution to 1 L.

Step 1: Convert the percentages to grams: 8% w/v = 8 g/100 ml.

Step 2: Set up a ratio/proportion problem: 1 L (1000 ml) is being made:

$$\frac{8g}{100\ ml} = \frac{X\ g}{1000\ ml}$$

Cross-multiply and divide. $X = 80$ g.

Step 3: Convert the other percentages the same way and tabulate them:

Calamine	80 g
Zinc oxide	80 g
Glycerol	20 g
Bentonite	250 g

q.s. with 2% calcium hydroxide solution to 1 L.

Making Solutions by Percentage

On occasion, a technician might be required to make a simple salt or drug solution by percentage. This simply involves calculating the amount of salt and adding the water.

Example: Prepare 2 L of saline (0.9% NaCl).

Step 1: Set up the ratio/proportion:

$$\frac{0.9\ g}{100\ ml} = \frac{X\ g}{2000\ ml}$$

Cross-multiply and divide. $X = 18$ g.

Step 2: Add 18 g of sodium chloride to 2 L of water.

Problems for Practice

Consider the following procedure for making a bulk laxative:

Psyllium	500 g
Dextrose	487.5 g
Citric acid	1 g
Sodium bicarbonate	1 g
Lemon flavoring	0.5 g
To make 1000 g	

Problems 1-5 relate to this procedure.

1. What is the percentage of psyllium in the preparation?
2. We need to make 5 kg of laxative. We have 10 g of citric acid. Do we have enough?
3. We want to make 500 g of laxative. How much psyllium do we need?
4. What is the percentage of bicarbonate in the preparation?
5. How much of each ingredient would be necessary to make 250 g of laxative?

Consider the following procedure for calamine lotion with antihistamine:

Calamine	80 g
Zinc oxide	80 g
Glycerol	20 g
Bentonite	245 g
Diphenhydramine	5 g
q.s. with 2% calcium hydroxide solution to 1 L.	

Problems 6-10 relate to this procedure.

6. What percentage of antihistamine is added?
7. How much diphenhydramine is needed to make 5 L of lotion?
8. How much lotion can we make with 60 g of zinc oxide?
9. How much glycerol is needed to make 240 ml of lotion?
10. If the ingredients in the preparation take up a volume of 50 ml, the total amount of calcium hydroxide added to the preparation would be:
    1. 1 L
    2. 850 ml
    3. 950 ml
    4. 1000 ml
11. We need 200 ml of a 2% solution of calcium hydroxide. How much calcium hydroxide do we need?
    1. 5 g
    2. 2.5 g
    3. 4 g
    4. 8 g

Solutions to Problems for Practice

1. The procedure calls for 500 g of psyllium and makes 1000 g.
   500 g/1000 g = **50%**.

2. The procedure calls for 1 g of citric acid to make 1 kg of laxative. Using ratio/proportion:

$$\frac{1\,g}{1\,kg} = \frac{X\,g}{5\,kg}$$

   Cross-multiply and divide: $X = 5$ g. We have 10 g. **Yes**.

3. The procedure makes 1000 g using 500 g of psyllium. Using ratio/proportion:

$$\frac{500\,g}{1000\,g} = \frac{X\,g}{500\,g}$$

   Cross-multiply and divide: $X =$ **250 g.**

4. The procedure calls for 1 g of bicarbonate to make 1000 g of laxative:

$$100\% \times \frac{1\,g}{1000\,g} = \mathbf{0.1\%}$$

5. Do the problem by ratio proportion, as in Problem 3. Calculate the amount of each ingredient as follows:

$$\frac{\text{amount specified in the procedure}}{1000\,g} = \frac{X}{250\,g}$$

   The reduced amounts correctly calculated will look like this:

Psyllium	125 g
Dextrose	121.9 g
Citric acid	0.25 g
Sodium bicarbonate	0.25 g
Lemon flavoring	0.125 g
To make 250 g	

6. Percentage is g/100 ml.

$$\frac{5\,g}{1000\,ml} = \frac{0.5\,g}{100\,ml} = \mathbf{0.5\%}.$$

7. The procedure makes 1 L, so we must multiply by 5 L/1 L, or 5. We need 5 g × 5 = **25 g.**

8. The procedure calls for 80 g, so 60 g ÷ 80 g × 1 L = **0.75 L**, or 750 ml.

9. (240 ml/1000 ml) × 20 g = **4.8 g.**

10. We q.s. to 1000 ml, so if the ingredients take up 50 ml of volume, we are actually adding 1000 ml – 50 ml = **950 ml** of calcium hydroxide solution. The correct answer is **3.**

11. Use ratio/proportion:

$$\frac{2\,g}{100\,ml} = \frac{X\,g}{200\,ml}$$

   Cross-multiply and divide: $X = 4$ g. The correct answer is **3.**

Chapter 22

Math Test with Solutions

The following questions will test your ability to answer mathematical questions in a multiple-choice format.

1. A milliliter is:
    1. 1/1000 of a liter.
    2. a unit of weight.
    3. a unit of volume.
    4. both 1 and 3 are correct.

2. Which of the following is not written correctly?
    1. 1.5 ml
    2. .5 ml
    3. 3/2 ml
    4. 1 1/2 ml
    5. both 2 and 3.

3. 50 ml =
    1. 0.5 L.
    2. 50000 mcl.
    3. 0.05 L.
    4. 0.005 L.
    5. both 2 and 3.

4. 10% of 50 g =
    1. 500 mg.
    2. 5000 mg.
    3. 0.5 mg.
    4. 5 g.
    5. both 2 and 4.

5. On a written prescription, gr xii would mean:
    1. 5 g
    2. 22 g
    3. 8 grains
    4. 12 grains

6. The instructions "one gtt A.U. qod" would be transcribed:
    1. 1 gram by mouth twice a day.
    2. place one drop in either eye every day.
    3. place one drop in each ear every other day.
    4. place one drop in both ears every other day.

7. You receive a box of gold. You would prefer it to weigh:
   1. 5 grams
   2. 5 grains
   3. 1 scruple
   4. 1 milligram

8. Which of the following is the smallest amount?
   1. 1 dram
   2. 1 scruple
   3. 1 teaspoon
   4. 5 milliliters

9. You receive an order for 25 units of U-100 insulin. Which of the following could not be dispensed ?
   1. A low-dose insulin syringe, containing 0.25 ml
   2. A low-dose insulin syringe, containing 25 U of U-100 insulin
   3. A U-100 syringe, containing 25 U of insulin
   4. A tuberculin syringe, containing 25 mcl of U-100 insulin
   5. either 2 or 3 would be acceptable, under appropriate conditions.

10. A prescription drug order reads "diazepam 2.5 mg IM bid." Available stock is in sealed 1 ml ampules containing 5 mg/ml. A unit dose would be:
    1. one ampule.
    2. two ampules.
    3. 5 ml.
    4. 10 ml in a 10 ml syringe.

11. You have an order for "codeine gr i tid prn." You have 30 mg tablets in stock. The label on the dispensing bottle should read:
    1. take one tablet twice a day.
    2. take two tablets twice a day.
    3. take two tablets three times a day.
    4. none of the above—the prescription must be filled exactly as written.

12. A patient is to take 15 ml of elixir twice a day. You would label the bottle with instructions to take _____ twice a day.
    1. 1 teaspoon
    2. 1 tablespoon
    3. 1 dram
    4. 3 teaspoon
    5. either 2 or 4

13. gr ss = _____ mg.
    1. 5
    2. 15
    3. 30
    4. 60

14. ℥ i =
    1. 20 ml.
    2. 5 ml.
    3. 15 ml.
    4. 30 ml.

15. 500 cc =
    1. 0.5 L.
    2. 500 ml.
    3. the volume contained in a cube with dimensions of 1 cm per side.
    4. all of the above.
    5. 1 and 2 only.

16. You are having a meal at 1300 hours. You are having:
    1. breakfast.
    2. lunch.
    3. dinner.
    4. a late-night snack.

17. A patient has a temperature of 37°C. If normal temperature is 98.6°F, he
    1. is cold.
    2. has a fever.
    3. is perfectly normal.
    4. is sick.

18. A parenteral drug is:
    1. placed in the eye.
    2. given by injection.
    3. placed on the skin.
    4. taken orally.
    5. given by suppository.

19. To reconstitute a drug you would:
    1. add a second drug to it.
    2. add water to it.
    3. dilute a solution.
    4. none of the above.

20. Your order is for cefoperazone 250 mg bid. Your stock is CefoBid suspension, 100 mg/ml. For a single dose, you would dispense:
    1. 5 ml.
    2. 10 ml.
    3. 2.5 ml.
    4. 0.5 ml.

21. For a *unit* dose of the prescription in Problem 20, you would dispense:
    1. 2.5 ml.
    2. 5 ml.
    3. 10 ml.
    4. 8 ml.

22. A 10% solution would be:
    1. 10 g/100 ml.
    2. 100 g/L.
    3. 100 mg/10 ml.
    4. 10 mg/ml.
    5. 1 and 2.

23. The order "Valium 20 mg IM stat" means to deliver:
    1. one tablet of Valium right now.
    2. 10 ml of Valium as soon as possible.
    3. an injection of 20 mg of Valium immediately.
    4. 20 ml of Valium in a dosage cup right away.

24. Your order is for morphine gr i. Available stock is 20 mg/ml. You dispense:
    1. 0.3 ml in a 1 ml syringe.
    2. 3 ml in a 3 ml syringe.
    3. 0.6 ml in a 1 ml syringe.
    4. 1.5 ml in a 3 ml syringe.

25. Your order is for furosemide 80 mg bid po. Your stock is Lasix 40 mg tablets. You dispense
    1. two tablets per dose.
    2. 1/2 tablet per dose.
    3. four tablets per unit dose.
    4. both 1 and 3.

26. A drug order is for nafcillin 0.25 g. In stock are 250 mg tablets. Dispense:
    1. four tablets.
    2. two tablets.
    3. one tablet.
    4. ten tablets.

27. 1 tab qid could mean:
    1. take one tablet twice a day.
    2. take one tablet four times a day.
    3. take one tablet every 6 hr.
    4. both 2 and 3.

28. 3 ml could not be accurately measured in:
    1. an oral syringe.
    2. a syringe for injection.
    3. a calibrated spoon.
    4. a dosage cup.

29. An insulin syringe:
    1. holds 1 ml.
    2. is calibrated in units.
    3. is the same as a tuberculin syringe.
    4. all of the above.
    5. 1 and 2.

30. 20 ml of a 10% solution contains____ g of drug.
    1. 200
    2. 20
    3. 2
    4. 0.2

31. The instructions on a prescription include the notation "1gtt OD am hs." The drug would be placed into the:
    1. right eye twice a day.
    2. left eye three times a day.
    3. right eye in the morning and evening.
    4. right eye in the morning and at bedtime.

Match the following to the correct description

A. dosage strength
B. dosage form
C. supply dosage

____ 32. a tablet

____ 33. a capsule

____ 34. 10 mg

____ 35. 10 mg/tablet

____ 36. parenteral solution

____ 37. 10000 U/10 ml

____ 38. 20% solution

____ 39. 10000 U

____ 40. tincture

____ 41. syrup

42. Your order is for 2000 ml of D_5W to run for 12 hours. The drop factor is 10 gtt/ml. The flow rate in gtt/min is:
    1. 12.
    2. 14.
    3. 28.
    4. 17.

43. Your order is 500 ml NS to run for 5 hours. The drop factor is 60 gtt/ml. The flow rate is ____ ml/min and ____ gtt/min.
    1. 0.8, 50
    2. 1.67, 100
    3. 1.8, 150
    4. 0.4, 24

44. You have an order for 75000 U of heparin to be infused over 4 hours. The 1 L bag contains 150,000 U of heparin. The flow rate needed to deliver the order is:
    1. 200 ml/hr.
    2. 150 ml/hr.
    3. 125 ml/hr.
    4. 100 ml/hr.

45. The recommended child dose of Keflex is 25 mg/kg/day in two divided doses. If a child weighs 66 lb, what is the correct dose?
    1. 375 mg bid
    2. 750 mg bid
    3. 700 mg qd
    4. 412 mg bid

46. The prescribed dose of drug for a child is 10 mg/m^2. His BSA is 0.8 m^2. The order would call for:
    1. 80 mg of drug.
    2. 0.08 mg of drug.
    3. 8 mg of drug.
    4. 47 mg of drug.

47. An IV bag containing a 2% solution of drug is running at 100 ml/hr. The hourly dose is:
    1. 20 mg.
    2. 200 mg.
    3. 2 g.
    4. 2 mg.

48. An order is for penicillin, to be infused at 100,000 U/hr. A 1 L IV bag containing 1,000,000 units of penicillin is used. The flow rate should be:
    1. 5 ml/min.
    2. 50 ml/hr.
    3. 100 ml/hr.
    4. 2 ml/min.

49. An adult dose of cefaclor is 6 mg/kg. The dose for a 66 lb child would be:
    1. 50 mg
    2. 180 mg
    3. 105.9 mg
    4. 198 mg

50. The child in Problem 49 is eight years old. Using Young's rule, the dose would be
    1. 79 mg.
    2. 174 mg.
    3. 72 mg.
    4. 80 mg.

51. The adult dose of a drug is 40 mg/kg. A child weighs 62 pounds. The child's dose would be:
    1. 240 mg.
    2. 663 mg.
    3. 1127 mg.
    4. 100 mg bid.

52. The adult dose of a drug is 100 mg. The dose for a child weighing 50 pounds would be:
    1. 75 mg.
    2. 50 mg.
    3. 150 mg.
    4. 25 mg.

53. A ten-year-old child receives the drug in #52. The dose prescribed would be:
    1. 50 mg.
    2. 75.2 mg.
    3. 45.45 mg.
    4. 30.6 mg.

54. Your order is for 2000 ml of D_5W to run for 12 hours. The flow rate in ml/min would be:
    1. 10 ml/min.
    2. 12 ml/min.
    3. 5 ml/min.
    4. 2.8 ml/min.

55. Your order is for 500 ml of NS to run for 4 hours. Your infusion set is labeled 10 gtt/ml. The flow rate in gtt/min would be:
    1. 2 gtt/min.
    2. 20.8 gtt/min.
    3. 21 gtt/min.
    4. 60 gtt/min.

56. Your order is for 75000 U of heparin to be infused over 8 hours. Available is a 1 L bag containing 100,000 U of heparin. The flow rate should be:
    1. 50 ml/hr.
    2. 100 ml/hr.
    3. 94 ml/hr.
    4. 45.2 ml/hr.

57. 100,000 U of penicillin is infused in 5 hours. The hourly dose would be:
    1. 10000 U.
    2. 20000 U.
    3. 50000 U.
    4. cannot be calculated from the information given.

58. A patient recieves D_5W at a rate of 100 ml/hr. The amount of dextrose administered per hour is:
    1. 50 mg.
    2. 1 g.
    3. 50 g.
    4. 5 g.

59. A patient receives 500 ml of a 1% calcium gluconate solution in 2 hours. The rate of infusion of calcium is
    1. 50 mg/min.
    2. 200 mg/hr.
    3. 1.5 g/hr.
    4. 41.7 mg/min.

60. The recommended child dose of Keflex is 25 mg/kg/day, in two divided doses. If a child weighs 73 lb, how much drug would be prescribed for one dose?
    1. 825 mg.
    2. 415 mg.
    3. 375 mg.
    4. 500 mg.

Solutions to Math Test

1. **4**
2. **5**
3. 50 ml × 1 L/1000 ml = 0.05 L = 50000 mcl. **3.**
4. 50 g = 50000 mg, so 10% (0.1) × 50 g = either 5 g or 5000 mg. **5.**
5. **4**
6. gtt = drop, A = ear, U = each, qod = every other day. **3.**
7. The largest amount is 5 g. **1.**
8. The smallest is 3 i, which is 4 ml. **1.**
9. You may use a 1 ml syringe with appropriate conversion, in an emergency. **1.**
10. Order: 2.5 mg. Stock: 5 mg/ml. 2.5 mg ÷ 5 mg/ml = 0.5 ml/*dose*. Unit dose = 1 ml. **1.**
11. gr i = 60 mg. **3.**
12. 15 ml = 1 T or 3 tsp. **5.**
13. ss = 1/2, so gr ss = 60 mg/2 = 30 mg. **3.**
14. **4.**
15. **5.**
16. **2.**
17. **3.**
18. **2.**
19. **2.**
20. **3.**
21. 2.5 ml × two times a day = 5 ml. **2.**
22. both 1 and 2. 1: 10 g/100 ml = 10%. 2: 100 g/L = 100 g/1000 ml = 10 g/100 ml = 10%. **5.**
23. **3.**
24. 60 mg × 20 mg/ml = 3 ml. **2.**
25. **4.**
26. **3.**
27. **4.**
28. **4.**
29. **5.**
30. 20 ml × 10 g/100 ml = 2 g. **3.**
31. **4.**

For problems 32–41, *dose* is in mg, g, etc. The *form* is the tablet, syrup, etc. *Supply dose* is mg/tablet, mg/ml, etc.

32. **B**		37. **C**	
33. **B**		38. **C**	
34. **A**		39. **A**	
35. **C**		40. **B**	
36. **B**		41. **B**	

42. First, calculate flow rate in ml/min: 2000 ml is infused in 12 hr (720 min). 2000 ml/720 min = 2.78 ml/min. Next, multiply by the drop factor: 2.78 ml/min × 10 gtt/ml = 27.8. Since you cannot have part of a drop, the answer is 28 gtt/min. **3.**

43. See Problem 42. **2.**

44. $C \times F = D/t$, so $F = D/t \div C$. D/t = 75000 U/4 hr, C = 150,000 U/1000 ml = 150 U/ml. 75000 U/4 hr = 18,750 U/hr. F = 18,750 U/hr ÷ 150 U/ml = 125 ml/hr. **3.**

45. 66 lb ÷ 2.2 lb/kg = 30 kg body weight. Dose = 25 mg/kg ÷ 30 kg = 750 mg/day. In two doses, each is 375 mg. **1.**

46. 10 mg/m^2 × 0.8 m^2 = 8 mg. **3.**

47. 2% = 2 g/100 ml. 2 g/100 ml × 100 ml/hr = 2 g. **3.**

48. See Problem 44. *D/t* = 100,000 U/hr, C = 1,000,000 U/1000 ml = 1000U/ml, F=100 ml/h. **3.**

49. 66 lb = 30 kg. 6 mg/kg × 30 kg = 180 mg adult dose. 180 mg/1.7 = child dose = 105.9 mg. **3.**

50. The adult dose is 180 mg. Child dose = [8years/(8 + 12)years] × 180 mg = 72 mg. **3.**

51. 62 lb = 28.18 kg. 40 mg/kg × 28.18 kg = 1127.27 mg (adult dose). 1127.27 mg/1.7 = 663 mg. **2.**

52. Use Clark's rule. 100 mg × 50/(150+50) = 25 mg. **4.**

53. Use Young's Rule: 100 mg × 10/(10 + 12) = 45.45 mg. **3.**

54. 12 hr = 720 min. 2000 ml/720 min = 2.79 ml/min. **4.**

55. **3.** See Problem 42.

56. C = 100,000 U/1000 ml = 100 U/ml. 75000 U/100 U/ml = 750 ml used in 8 hr = 94 ml/hr. **3.**

57. 100,000 U/5 hr = 20000 U/hr. **2.**

58. D$_5$W is 5% dextrose. 5000 mg/100 ml = 50 mg/ml concentration. 50 mg/ml × 100 ml/hr = 5 g. **4.**

59. 1% = 1000 mg/100 ml = 10 mg/ml. 10 mg/ml × 500 ml = 5000 mg infused in 2 hr = 2500 mg/hr. 2500 mg/hr × 1 hr/60 min = 41.67 mg/min. **4.**

60. 73 lb = 33.2 kg. 33.2 kg × 25 mg/kg/day = 830 mg/day. In two doses, 415 mg/dose. **2.**

Pharmacy Operations

Chapter 23   Safety in the Workplace

Chapter 24   Using Computers in the Pharmacy

Chapter 25   Communications Within the Pharmacy

Safety in the Workplace

Quick Study

(See text for full explanation.)

I. **Occupational Safety and Health Administration (OSHA)**

   A. *Safety guidelines:*

- Floors must be clean and dry
- Floors/aisles and counters should be free of clutter
- Exits and fire doors should be clearly marked and accessible
- Sharp objects and hazardous materials should be properly stored when not in use
- OSHA approved personal protection must be worn when working with hazardous materials

II. **Disposal of hazardous waste**

   A. *Sharps and needles*

   B. *Hazardous chemicals* (i.e., chemotherapeutic drugs, steroids, etc.)

III. **Cleaning spills of hazardous materials**

   A. Mercury and toxic materials

   B. Flammable substances

Occupational Health and Safety Administration Regulations

Work within the pharmacy is required to be conducted in a safe, sanitary manner, in order to protect the health and safety of the patient. However, additional safeguards must be followed to protect the health and safety of the pharmacy personnel.

The Occupational Health and Safety Administration (OSHA) was designed to protect employees in the workplace. OSHA has standards of safety and sanitation that must be met. It conducts periodic site visits or inspections to ensure that the pharmacy and its employees are working within appropriate safety guidelines (compliance).

OSHA regulations state that:

- The floors in the work area must be clean and dry. This regulation is designed to help avoid accidents like slipping on wet floors, or floors that have grit, dust, or other contaminants on the surface.

- The pharmacy aisle should be free of boxes or other clutter. Again, this regulation helps to prevent accidents, such as tripping over boxes, or knocking materials off of the pharmacy bench, while trying to avoid the boxes.

- The exits and fire doors should be clearly marked and accessible — no boxes, barrels, or equipment should block exits.

- Sharp objects and utensils should be put away when not in use. This includes sharps and needles as well as small spatulas, which could cause injury should they flip off the bench and land on a foot, on a hand, or in an eye.

- Flammable or caustic substances should be properly stored when not in use. They should not be left on the pharmacy bench. Flammable substances should be stored in specially vented "flammable" cabinets, or, if necessary, in an explosion-proof refrigerator.

- OSHA-approved personal protective equipment should be worn when working with hazardous chemicals or drugs. This may include safety glasses and goggles. Closed-toe shoes and clothing that covers the arms and legs should also be worn.

In addition:

- Acids and bases, such as hydrochloric acid and sodium hydroxide, should never be stored in the same cabinet. If the two were to mix, a violent reaction would occur.

Disposal of Hazardous Waste

Hazardous waste includes needles, syringes, and toxic chemicals (drugs). Needles or syringes should never be thrown in the trash. Sharps and needles can pose a health hazard to anyone using or disposing of the trash and could wind up in landfills or other public places (such as lakes or beaches, should the hospital's disposal company be so sloppy). Syringes can be re-used by unauthorized persons, if found in the trash. To avoid this, both needles and syringes should be placed into an autoclavable sharps container for autoclaving (high heat treatment) and disposal.

Toxic substances, especially those such as cancer chemotherapeutics, should never be disposed of through the regular trash or by pouring the material down the drain, because this would contaminate the water supply of the area. Instead, these substances should be placed into a **biohazard bag** for destruction.

Sanitation Management

Obvious cleanliness procedures should always be followed: rinsing or washing equipment for liquid measure and wiping off dispensing trays and tablet counters before and after each use. Whenever a device is used for measure, there is always some residue of drug, however small, remaining on the surface of the device. If the device is used again without proper cleaning, this residue may be incorporated into the new prescription, causing cross contamination of drugs, which should be avoided.

Spills

Procedures must exist for the proper cleanup of substances spilled in the work area. Many substances used within a pharmacy are toxic, not only drugs (especially antineoplastics) but other substances as well, such as phenol and mercury (e.g., from a broken thermometer).

Flammable Materials

Spills of flammable materials, such as alcohol, should first be contained so that the material does not contact electrical outlets on the floor or bench. Since it is the fumes (vapors) that ignite, proper ventilation must be provided. Electrical appliances such as portable fans should not be used for this purpose, due to sparks, which could ignite the fumes. After containment, an absorbent material is placed on the spill, and, once absorbed, the material is swept away and disposed of in a well-ventilated area.

Acids, Bases, or Caustic Materials

Acids and bases are dangerous because they can dissolve most materials, including human skin (indeed, caustics like phenol are used to dissolve calluses on the feet and cauterize wounds). If an acid or basic substance is spilled, it must first be neutralized before the spill is cleaned. When the opposite substance is added (i.e., a weak acid to neutralize a base), the spilled substance becomes a salt, which is not hazardous to clean or dispose of. However, because of the potential of a strong chemical reaction, only weak acids or bases should be used to neutralize, such as acetic acid or sodium bicarbonate. Mixing a strong acid and base would produce a violent chemical reaction and possibly an explosion. Once neutralized, the substance can be cleaned with disposable towels or wipes and thrown in the paper trash or may be disposed of down the drain.

Mercury

Mercury is an extremely toxic substance — it is a "heavy metal," and one of the few substances that is eliminated from the body so slowly as to essentially not be eliminated at all. Mercury, at room temperature, exists in a liquid form and so goes directly into a vapor ("sublimation"). If mercury is spilled, it can be inhaled through the respiratory tract as well as absorbed through the skin. Thus, it is essential that these spills be cleaned up immediately. A spill kit is used that contains a porous sponge (to trap the small spheres of mercury and prevent dissemination throughout the area). The sponge should be used in a gentle blotting motion to avoid breaking up the spheres into smaller spheres, thus increasing the probability of sublimation. Mercury also reacts very quickly with gold, so remove any jewelry before attempting to clean a mercury spill.

Antineoplastic Drugs

Safety precautions for working with antineoplastic drugs were discussed in Chapter 4. Similar precautions should be used when cleaning spills of antineoplastic drugs or other potentially hazardous drugs.

Spills of antineoplastic drugs should be cleaned according to proper procedure and disposed of properly. Should the spill come in contact with a person, the drug should be brushed from the skin (if it is in powder form) and removed as much as possible *before* washing thoroughly, to prevent absorption of the drug through the skin. If the spill is in liquid form, care must be taken not to rub the affected area, which would drive the drug into the skin. Liquid drug on the surface of the skin should be gently blotted off before the skin is washed thoroughly. Affected clothing should be removed immediately. It is also wise to wear a mask, goggles, and gloves when cleaning a spill.

Regardless of spillage, when working with these drugs, one must be careful never to touch the area around the eyes, nose, or mouth. Working with gloves may protect the hands from exposure but will not prevent the drug from entering the body if the contaminated gloved hands come in contact with the mucous membranes of the eyes, nose, or mouth. Reflex actions of rubbing an itching eye or nose should be avoided.

Questions for Review

1. OSHA exists to protect the health and safety of the:
   1. patient.
   2. administration.
   3. worker.
   4. worker within the pharmacy.

2. Which is the best way to dispose of a syringe and needle?
   1. Cut both the syringe barrel and needle in half and discard.
   2. Place both syringe and needle in an autoclavable sharps container.
   3. Cut the needle off of the syringe and discard.
   4. Place both syringe and needle in a biohazard (red) bag.

3. When working with antineoplastic (anticancer) drugs, one should wear:
   1. clothing that has long sleeves and covers the legs.
   2. a protective cloth coat.
   3. a paper coat, hat, shoe covers, and goggles.
   4. any of the above.
   5. 1 and 3.

4. The first step in cleaning an alcohol spill should be
   1. absorbing the material.
   2. protecting exposed electrical outlets.
   3. turning off any open flames or electrical appliances.
   4. using paper towels to wipe up the spill.
   5. both 2 and 3.

5. All areas of the workplace must be:
   1. dry.
   2. free of dirt and dust.
   3. clean.
   4. 1, 2, and 3.

6. When dealing with a spill of a toxic drug on your skin you should:
   1. immediately place the area under running water.
   2. scrub the affected area.
   3. gently blot the drug solution from the area with an absorbent towel before washing.
   4. wash the area with soap and water.

7. The first step in cleaning a spill of hydrochloric acid might be:
   1. washing with water.
   2. absorbing the material with paper towels.
   3. placing some sodium bicarbonate on top of the spilled material.
   4. using a sponge to clean the spill.

8. Wearing protective clothing and gloves is sufficient to protect the worker from the toxic effects of antineoplastic drugs unless
   1. the gloves are too thin.
   2. the sleeves on the coat are too long.
   3. the worker rubs his or her eyes or nose while working.
   4. the worker is working too close to the drug material.

Solutions to Questions for Review

1. OSHA was designed to protect the worker, not the patient or administration. The correct answer is **3**.

2. Because of the risk of infection, all sharps, needles, and syringes are placed in an autoclavable sharps container and autoclaved at high temperatures before disposal. The correct answer is **2**.

3. When working with these drugs, disposable outer clothing (gowns, hats, gloves, shoe covers) should be worn, not cloth coats that have to be washed and would contaminate the water supply. All exposed parts of the body should be covered as well. The correct answer is **5**.

4. With a spill of flammable material, always extinguish flames and turn off appliances immediately; however, barricading outlets is equally important. The correct answer is **5**.

5. 1, 2, and 3 are all correct. The correct answer is **4**.

6. Never rub skin that has been contaminated with drug. Always blot or brush the drug off before washing. The correct answer is **3**.

7. Before cleaning a caustic spill, first neutralize the material. The correct answer is **3**.

8. Protective clothing is no protection if a worker rubs his or her eye, mouth, or nose with clothing contaminated with the drug. The correct answer is **3**.

Chapter 24

Using Computers in the Pharmacy

Quick Study

(See text for full explanation.)

I. **Uses of computers**

    A. *Repetitive tasks* such as inventory, billing, pricing, maintenance of patient records

    B. *Education* of pharmacy personnel

    C. Assistance in procedures for *preparation of drug products*

    D. General *communication*

II. **Components of a computer and their functions**

    A. *Hardware*

        • Memory storage units and circuitry—the central processing unit (CPU) and fixed ('hard') disc

        • Peripheral units (printer, monitor, etc.)

    B. *Software*

        • A set of instructions for the computer to follow

        • Information stored on floppy discs and installed onto the hard disc

III. **Input devices feed information into the computer:**

    A. Light pen, optical scanner, keyboard

IV. **Output devices export information from the computer**

    A. Monitor, printer, modem, etc.

V. **Information storage**

    A. *Permanent storage* in 'bits' and 'bytes' (*read-only memory ROM*)

        • CD ROM

        • Fixed disc

        • Floppy disc

    B. *Temporary storage: random access memory (RAM)*

Use of Computers in Pharmacy Practice

Computers are almost indispensable in the pharmacy. Using computers we can keep track of drug inventory, narcotics use, changes in the drug formulary, and personnel. Computers are used for patient billing, insurance billing and verification, pricing, maintenance of patient profiles, generation of the medication administration record, and a number of computational and repetitive tasks.

Education of Pharmacy Personnel

Computers are useful in the education of pharmacy personnel. Since drug products change rapidly, as do developments in physiology, biochemistry, and pharmacology, constant education and review are necessary for the competent practice of pharmacy. Computers can provide the pharmacist or technician with information on a particular topic, references, communication with researchers and pharmaceutical companies, and the like.

Computers in Clinical Practice

A properly programmed computer may suggest the proper diluting agent (diluent) to use in preparing an IV (some drugs are more compatible with a particular diluent, e.g., NS as opposed to water, or D_5W as opposed to NS, etc.), and the computer may even suggest a procedure for dilution or compounding. Computer programs may also alert the pharmacist to potential drug-drug interactions and drug-physiology interactions, to safeguard the patient.

Communication by Computer

Computers are useful in communication (see Chapter 25 and Chapters 1–3) from the prescriber to the pharmacy and vice-versa. They may also be useful in obtaining information related to a patient or a patient's condition from poison control centers, research centers, and other organizations that are highly computerized.

The Components of a Computer

The working computer consists of two main divisions: **hardware** and **software**. The hardware is the circuitry, storage units, and peripheral ("add-on") units of the computer, whereas the software is a set of instructions for the computer to follow enabling it to perform a specific function. The software is usually stored on floppy discs and installed onto the hardware (hard drive). The hardware portions of the computer consist of the following:

- The **central processing unit (CPU)** is a compact unit that contains the computer's memory, components used in data storage (such as the fixed, or hard, disk and memory chips), communication (the modem), and sound generation; and, most importantly, the unit that processes the data before displaying it on the monitor screen or printer. The CPU may connect with a floppy (peripheral) disk drive which writes to a removable floppy disk for additional data storage.

- The monitor is a "television set" that allows the operator to see data and information displayed by the computer. This is an **output device**, meaning that information from the computer goes *out* to the device to be displayed for the user.

- The **printer** is an output device that allows information to be printed out as a hard copy rather than viewed on a screen.

- The **light pen** and **optical scanner** are two **input devices** that carry information to the computer. This information is used by the computer to calculate charges, access information, and so forth. These devices are able to "read" bar-coded information on drug packaging and relay it to the computer's processor. The **keyboard** is another example of an input device, where information is typed in by the user for the computer to process.

Storage of Information

Information may be *permanently* stored on the fixed disk, a small, flat disc of hard plastic that contains grooves, much like a record. The more grooves that the disc has and the closer together they are, the more capacity the disc has to store information. Storage area is measured in **bits**, which are grouped into larger **bytes**. A *kilo*byte is 1000 bytes, a *mega*byte is 1,000,000 bytes, and a *giga*byte is 100,000,000 bytes. The floppy disc is similar but is able to store less information. Both types of discs must be formatted by the disc operating system software before they can be used with the system. Formatting prepares the disc to be used and also erases any information already stored on the disc

Information may be temporarily stored in the computer's memory, or **buffer**. When you are working on the computer, the computer program in use as well as the information entered into the computer are all stored in the buffer. This is why, if the computer loses power or is shut off, information that was entered but not saved to disk is lost.

Memory

There are two types of memory: **read only memory (ROM)** and **random access memory (RAM)**. A disc that is protected, so that it cannot be written on (no data can be stored on it), is only able to show information—the information cannot be erased or destroyed by formatting. This information goes to the computer in a specific sequence which tells the computer what to do. An example of ROM would be a compact disc (CD) used for storing information. The hard disc has ROM but is able to accept information for storage as well.

Random access memory (RAM) is found in the computer or printer buffer, where data is temporarily stored. Movement of this information into the buffer is defined by the user. Storage of data is temporary, and the information contained in it must be permanently stored or will be lost when the power supply is interrupted or turned off.

Questions for Review

1. Temporary storage of data occurs in the:
   1. random access memory.
   2. disk operating system.
   3. read only memory.
   4. buffered memory.

2. Which of the following is not an output device?
   1. Monitor
   2. Printer
   3. Optical scanner
   4. Plotter

3. Which of the following is not considered computer hardware?
   1. Hard disc
   2. Modem
   3. Processor
   4. Disk operating system

4. Which of the following is not a use for computers in the pharmacy?
   1. Maintaining patient information
   2. Billing
   3. Generating prescriptions
   4. Identifying drug-drug interactions

5. An example of an input device would be a:
   1. light pen.
   2. printer.
   3. modem.
   4. monitor.

6. You generate a profile for a patient and save it in the RAM. You can retrieve the information later from the:
   1. hard disc.
   2. floppy disc.
   3. memory.
   4. The information cannot be retrieved.

Solutions to Questions for Review

1. Storage in random access memory is temporary. The correct answer is **1**.

2. Output goes from the computer to the user. This would include the monitor, printer, and graphics device (plotter), but an optical scanner sends information to the computer. The correct answer is **3**.

3. The disk operating system is a set of instructions for the computer that tells it what to do. The correct answer is **4**.

4. This is a trick question. Computers do not generate prescriptions, prescribers do. The correct answer is **3**.

5. All of these devices send information *out*, except for the light pen. The correct answer is **1**.

6. Information cannot be permanently saved in the random access memory. The next application would erase it from memory. The correct answer is **4**.

Chapter 25

Communications Within the Pharmacy

Quick Study

(See text for full explanation.)

I. **Role of the pharmacist**
   A. Patient consultation
   B. Medical advisement, recommendation of emergency procedures
   C. Receipt of prescriptions generated by electronic means
   D. Accepts refill authorizations

II. **Role of the technician**
   A. Communication regarding *routine requests*
   B. Communication with third party payers to verify payment
   C. Answering of general questions to limitations of knowledge
   D. Verification of prescription orders
   E. Providing support to the patient

What sort of communications exist within the pharmacy? The technician communicates with the patient, the pharmacist, other pharmacy personnel, nurses, physicians, and outside groups.

Role of the Technician in Communication

The technician may:

- Communicate with patients, prescribers, and caregivers regarding routine requests.
- Communicate with third-party payers to ensure payment to the pharmacy.

- Refer patients to the pharmacist for consultation. If the questions or potential problems that the patient may have regarding a medication or condition require advice and professional judgment, the patient *must* be referred to the pharmacist. The technician is not qualified to address these questions, and to do so may cause the pharmacist to lose his or her professional license.

- Clarify prescription orders with the prescriber, if necessary. If the prescription is illegible or the instructions ambiguous, the technician is allowed, at the discretion of the pharmacist, to clarify the prescription order with the prescriber.

- Communicate with other pharmacy personnel and technicians.

- Answer general questions about medication and dosing, to the limits of his or her knowledge, provided that the answers do not require any judgment by the technician.

- Offer support to the patient. This may include recommending reading material or other resources to patients, should they require it.

The technician may *not*:

- Offer advice to the patient regarding drug products.

- Counsel the patient in any way.

- Answer questions about drug interactions or physical interactions with a drug product.

- Recommend procedures of any kind, such as induction of vomiting with overdose, supplementary medication, etc.

- Take prescription orders electronically (i.e., from another computer [by modem] or by telephone).

- Take prescriptions or authorizations by telephone.

Role of the Pharmacist in Communication

The role of the pharmacist is to dispense advice, answer all questions or address all problems requiring professional judgment, and handle any emergency situations. Patients frequently call the pharmacy with questions about a drug which has been prescribed for them or an over the counter drug which they are taking. Occasionally, a patient may even call the pharmacy in an emergency (a child has taken the medication, for example, or the patient has overdosed) and ask what to do. These calls should *immediately* be referred to the pharmacist. Not all callers will be looking for information on a drug to be sure that they are using it properly; some callers will be looking for information which will allow them to select or obtain a drug for *abuse*. The pharmacist has the ability to screen these calls and dispense the proper advice. The technician is not trained to do so, and for the technician to dispense advice, however accurate, is technically illegal. The role of the technician *is* changing, however, with the advent of the national certification exam, formal training of technicians, and, in some states, licensure of technicians.

Questions for Review

1. A patient calls, saying that her young son has taken her medication by mistake and may have overdosed. You should:
    1. tell her to call 911.
    2. refer her to the nearest poison control center.
    3. attempt to comfort her.
    4. refer her to the pharmacist.
2. The technician is *not* allowed to
    1. call the prescriber to clarify a prescription order.
    2. offer support to the patient.
    3. tell the patient not to take aspirin with her Coumadin prescription.
    4. tell the patient that the pharmacy carries a generic drug for her prescription that is considerably cheaper than the proprietary drug.
3. A patient has a question about a drug you know a lot about. You should:
    1. answer her questions.
    2. refer her to the pharmacist.
    3. refer her to information in the library.
    4. tell her that you are not allowed to give out this information.
4. Communication between two computers over telephone lines is accomplished by the use of a:
    1. fax machine.
    2. printer.
    3. modem.
    4. computer monitor.

Solutions to Questions for Review

1. Emergency calls are always referred to the pharmacist. The correct answer is **4.**

2. The technician may not offer advice regarding drug-drug interactions. The correct answer is **3.**

3. It would be acceptable for the technician to provide source information (reading material) for the patient; however, the correct answer is to refer the patient to the pharmacist. The correct answer is **2.**

4. Communication from computer to computer is accomplished by the use of a *modem*. The correct answer is **3.**

Pharmacology

Chapter 26 Drug Nomenclature

Chapter 27 The Pharmacology of Drug Interactions

Drug Nomenclature

Quick Study

(See text for full explanation.)

I. **Proprietary drug names**
   A. As related to drug function
   B. As related to drug classification

II. **Knowledge of general therapeutic actions of drugs**

III. **Representative drugs, dosage forms, and strengths available**

Introduction

The PCTB exam, at the time of this writing, contains little of what is truly considered to be pharmacology, such as drug mechanisms of action; however, it is anticipated that this will change. The present PCTB examination tests on drug classifications, general uses, side effects, and interactions and will include both generic and proprietary names. Thus, a representative sampling of frequently prescribed drugs will be presented here along with a guide to the nomenclature (naming) of drugs, particularly the proprietary names. Attention should be paid, in this chapter and the following chapter, to the general therapeutic action of a particular drug, the class (tricyclic antidepressant, benzodiazepine, opiate, etc.), and the proprietary names for a particular generic drug, as well as the availability of particular dosage forms and strengths (e.g., 10 mg tablet).

Note that most drugs have been treated with an acid or base and thus are salts of the original drug. This has been done to make the drug easier to be absorbed and utilized by the body. These drugs may have words such as "mesylate", "tartrate", "citrate", or "hydrochloride (HCl)" after their names, or the words "sodium" or "potassium". Penicillin G potassium (Penicillin G-K) is the potassium salt of penicillin, for example. In a few cases, this addition means that a drug is used for a different purpose. For example, erythromycin gluceptate is used by parenteral route, erythromycin succinate is used orally, and erythromycin estolate is a highly absorbable form of erythromycin. The addition of the type of salt to the name of the drug is seldom used in practice especially if only one form of the drug exists. Drugs are simply referred to by name (e.g., trazadone, rather than trazadone hydrochloride).

Addition of letters to a drug name is usually important, however. For example, penicillin G is the form of penicillin normally given by parenteral route, while penicillin V is given orally. The addition of the letters "SR" after a drug name denote a sustained release formulation, and NPH (neutral protamine hagadorn) insulin is a complexed form of insulin which is longer acting.

Proprietary Drug Nomenclature

Drugs are named according to what they do, their drug classification, or less frequently, by some other property that they have, such as fast onset (Allegra) or long duration (Cardura) or dosing interval (Cefo*bid*). In many cases, the use and/or class of a drug can be determined from the name. For example, take the drug Tegopen. This drug is a penicillin derivative—the name ends in *pen*. The drug is actually cloxacillin. Many drugs simply take part of the generic name as the trade name, or contract the generic name; for instance, Amoxil is *amoxi*cillin, Buspar is *buspir*one, Platinol is cis*platin*, and Pilocar is *pilocar*pine. Most of the cephalosporin antibiotics have *cef* or something similar in the name, such as Cefobid, Keflex, Biocef, and Keftab. Most proprietary names are unimaginative, so if you are faced with a question on the exam and you are not familiar with the drug name, you can make an educated guess. (When working in the pharmacy it is, of course, better to use the "generic-to-brand" book. Unfortunately, you cannot bring it to the exam.)

The following pages list some frequently prescribed drugs. Both the generic and major proprietary names are stated; however, many drugs have several manufacturers, each with a different proprietary name for the drug. I have listed only two or three of the most commonly prescribed ones (major brand names). I have also included what type of a drug it is (its classification) and a brief description of the mechanism of action. (For basic information on therapies and drug mechanisms and interactions, see Chapter 27; for more in-depth information, see a good pharmacology text or drug reference.)

Look for the similarities between the proprietary names and the generic name, or the drug's function. This will help you recognize the name and associate it. Also, when memorizing names of drugs, it is very helpful to prepare flash cards. Some drugs can only be remembered by straight memorization; however, if you can recognize the similarities between drugs, name, and function, you will be able to recognize drugs that you may not have memorized.

If you are working in a pharmacy already, some drug names will be familiar to you. A pharmacology text or nurse's drug reference might be a source of drug names and classifications to memorize.

Drugs That Affect the Central Nervous System

Drugs Used for Depression

(Serotonin reuptake inhibitors are also used in the therapy of migraine headaches.)

tranylcypromine

Brand name: *Parnate*

Classification: monoamine oxidase inhibitor

Available as: 10 mg tablet

amitriptyline hydrochloride

Brand name: *Elavil*

Classification: tricyclic antidepressant

Available as: 10 mg, 25 mg, 50 mg, 75 mg, 100 mg, 150 mg tablets; and 10 mg/ml injection

nortriptyline hydrochloride

Brand names: *Aventyl*, *Pamelor*

Classification: tricyclic antidepressant

Available as: 10 mg, 25 mg, 50 mg, and 75 mg tablets; 10 mg/5 ml injection

amoxapine

Brand name: *Asendin*

Classification: heterocyclic antidepressant

Available as: 25 mg, 50 mg, 100 mg, and 150 mg tablets

bupropion

Brand name: *Wellbutrin*

Classification: heterocyclic antidepressant

Available as: 75 mg and 100 mg tablets

trazadone

Brand name: *Desyrel*

Classification: heterocyclic antidepressant

Available as: 50 mg, 100 mg, 150 mg, and 300 mg tablets

paroxetine hydrochloride

Brand name: *Paxil*

Classification: serotonin reuptake inhibitor

Available as: 10 mg, 20 mg, 30 mg, and 40 mg tablets

sertraline hydrochloride

Brand name: *Zoloft*

Classification: serotonin reuptake inhibitor

Available as: 50 mg and 100 mg tablets

sumatriptan succinate

Brand name: *Imitrex*

Classification: serotonin receptor (5 HT_1) agonist

Available as: 25 mg and 50 mg tablets; 1.6 mg/0.5 ml injection

venlafaxine hydrochloride

Brand name: *Effexor*

Classification: serotonin reuptake inhibitor

Available as: 25 mg, 37.5 mg, 50 mg, 75 mg, and 100 mg tablets

Drugs Used for Anxiety

buspirone hydrochloride

Brand name: *BuSpar*

Classification: Non-benzodiazepine antianxiety agent

Available as: 5 mg, 10 mg, and 15 mg tablets

alprazolam

Brand name: *Xanax*

Classification: benzodiazepine

Available as: 0.25 mg, 0.5 mg, 1 mg, and 2 mg tablets; 1 mg/ml concentrate; 0.5 mg/5 ml solution

lorazepam

Brand name: *Ativan*

Classification: benzodiazepine

Available as: 0.5 mg, 1 mg, and 2 mg tablets; 2 mg/ml concentrate; 2 mg/ml and 4 mg/ml injection

Drugs Used for Seizures

carbamazepine
Brand name: *Tegretol*
Classification: sodium channel blocker
Available as: 100 mg and 200 mg tablets

gabapentin
Brand name: *Neurontin*
Classification: analog of gamma aminobutyric acid (GABA)
Available as: 100 mg, 300 mg, and 400 mg capsules

lamotrigine
Brand name: *Lamictal*
Classification: antagonist of glutamate
Available as: 100 mg and 200 mg tablets

phenytoin (diphenylhydantoin)
Brand names: *Dilantin Infatab, Dilantin-125*
Classification: inhibitor of sodium/potassium conductance
Available as: 50 mg chewable tablet; 100 mg/4 ml and 125 mg/5 ml suspension

phenytoin sodium, extended
Brand name: *Dilantin Kapseals*
Classification: inhibitor of sodium/potassium conductance
Available as: 30 mg and 100 mg capsules

phenytoin sodium, parenteral
Brand name: *Dilantin Sodium*
Classification: inhibitor of sodium/potassium conductance
Available as: 50 mg/ml injection

phenytoin sodium prompt
Brand name: *Diphenylan Sodium*
Classification: inhibitor of sodium/potassium conductance
Available as: 100 mg capsule

valproic acid and derivatives

Brand names: *Depakene* (valproic acid), *Depakote* (divalproex sodium salt, sustained release)

Classification: potentiation of GABA levels/activity

Available as: 125 mg, 250 mg tablets; 500 mg sustained release tablets; 250 mg capsule; and 250 mg/ml syrup (sodium salt); 500 mg tablets (SR)

Drugs Used for Attention-Deficit Disorder

methylphenidate hydrochloride

Brand name: *Ritalin*

Classification: Central nervous system stimulant

Available as: 5 mg, 10 mg, and 20 mg tablets; 20 mg extended-release tablet

Drugs Used in the Therapy of Parkinson's Disease

bromocriptine mesylate

Brand name: *Parlodel*

Classification: dopaminergic agonist

Available as: 2.5 mg tablet; 5 mg capsule

levodopa

Brand names: *Dopar, Larodopa*

Classification: dopaminergic precursor

Available as: 100 mg, 250 mg, and 500 mg tablets and capsules

levodopa/carbidopa

Brand name: *Sinemet*

Classification: combination drug—dopaminergic precursor with enzyme inhibitor

Available as: 100 mg levodopa with 10 mg or 25 mg carbidopa tablets; 250 mg levodopa with 25 mg carbidopa tablet

Antipsychotic Drugs

clozapine

Brand name: *Clozaril*

Classification: antipsychotic

Available as: 25 mg, 100 mg tablets

fluphenazine

Brand name: *Permitil, Prolixin*

Classification: antipsychotic

Available as: 1 mg, 2.5 mg, 10 mg tablets; 2.5 mg/5 ml elixir; 5 mg/ml concentrate; 2.6 mg/ml IM injection

haloperidol

Brand name: *Haldol*

Classification: antipsychotic

Available as: 0.5 mg, 1 mg, 2 mg, 5 mg, 10 mg, 20 mg tablets; 2 mg/ml concentrate; 5 mg/ml solution for IM injection

loxapine hydrochloride

Brand name: *Loxitane*

Classification: antipsychotic

Available as: 5 mg, 10 mg, 25 mg, 50 mg capsules; 2 mg/ml concentrate; 5 mg/ml solution for IM injection

Centrally Acting Narcotics Used to Relieve Pain

codeine and acetaminophen

Brand name: *Tylenol #1, #2, #3, or #4*

Classification: narcotic analgesic with acetaminophen

Available as: 10 mg codeine (#1), 15 mg codeine (#2), 30 mg codeine (#3), or 60 mg codeine (#4), with 300 mg acetaminophen tablets

hydrocodone and acetaminophen

Brand names: *Anexia, Lorcet, Vicodin*

Classification: opiate narcotic (C II)

Available as: 5 mg/500 mg acetaminophen, 7.5 mg/650 mg and 10 mg/650 mg (Anexia), 10 mg/650 mg acetaminophen (Lorcet) tablets

hydromorphone hydrochloride

Brand name: *Dilaudid*

Classification: narcotic analgesic

Available as: 1 mg, 2 mg, 3 mg, and 4 mg tablets; 3 mg suppositories; 1 mg/ml, 2 mg/ml, 3 mg/ml, 4 mg/ml, and 10 mg/ml solution for injection

meperidine hydrochloride

Brand name: *Demerol*

Classification: narcotic analgesic

Available as: 50 mg, 100 mg tablets; 50 mg/5 ml oral suspension; 10 mg/ml, 50 mg/ml, and 100 mg/ml sterile solution for injection; 25 mg, 50 mg, 75 mg, and 100 mg dosettes

oxycodone hydrochloride

Brand names: *Percocet*, *Percodan*

Classification: narcotic analgesic with nonsteroidal analgesic

Available as: 4.9 mg oxycodone with 325 mg aspirin (Percodan); 5 mg oxycodone with 325 mg or 500 mg aspirin (Percocet)

propoxyphene hydrochloride with aspirin

Brand names: *Darvon, Doloxene, Progesic*

Classification: narcotic analgesic (C IV)

Available as: 65 mg capsules

propoxyphene napsylate

Brand name: *Darvon-N*

Classification: narcotic analgesic (C IV)

Available as: 100 mg tablet

Centrally Acting Non-Narcotic Drugs Used to Relieve Pain

tramadol hydrochloride

Brand name: *Ultram*

Classification: centrally acting analgesic

Available as: 50 mg tablet

Nonsteroidal Anti-inflammatory Drugs

ibuprofen

Major brand names: *IBU, Motrin, Advil*

Classification: nonsteriodal anti-inflammatory drug, cyclooxygenase inhibitor

Available as: 100 mg, 200 mg, 300 mg, 400 mg, 600 mg, and 800 mg tablets; 50 mg and 100 mg chewable tablets; 50 mg/1.25 ml and 100 mg/5 ml oral suspension

nabumetone

Brand name: *Relafen*

Classification: nonsteriodal anti-inflammatory drug (NSAID)

Available as: 500 mg and 750 mg tablets

naproxen

Brand names: *Naprosyn, EC-Naprosyn*

Classification: NSAID

Available as: 375 mg and 500 mg enteric coated tablets; 250 mg, 375 mg, and 500 mg tablets; 25 mg/ml suspension

naproxen sodium

Major brand names: *Anaprox, Naprelan*

Classification: NSAID

Available as: 220 mg, 275 mg, and 500 mg tablets; 375 mg and 500 mg extended-release tablets

Drugs That Affect the Cardiovascular System

These affect the heart, or vessels, or directly alter the activity of the autonomic nervous system.

Drugs Used for Hypertension

Note: Beta blockers and calcium channel blockers are also used in the therapy of angina.

amlodipine

Brand name: *Norvasc*

Classification: calcium channel blocker

Available as: 2.5 mg, 5 mg and 10 mg tablets

diltiazem hydrochloride

Major brand names: *Cardizem, Dilacor, Tiazac*

Classification: calcium channel blocker

Available as: 30 mg, 60 mg, 90 mg, and 120 mg tablets; 5 mg/ml solution for injection; 60 mg, 90 mg, 120 mg, 180 mg, 240 mg, 300 mg, and 360 mg extended-release capsules

nifedipine

Major brand names: *Adalat, Procardia, Procardia XL*

Classification: calcium channel blocker

Available as: 10 mg and 20 mg capsules; 30 mg, 60 mg, and 90 mg extended-release tablets

verapamil hydrochloride

Major brand names: *Calan, Isoptin, Verelan*

Classification: calcium channel blocker

Available as: 40 mg, 80 mg, and 120 mg tablets; 120 mg, 180 mg, and 240 mg extended-release tablets; 120 mg, 180 mg, 240 mg, and 360 mg extended release capsules; 2.5 mg/ml solution for injection

atenolol

Brand name: *Tenormin*

Classification: beta adrenergic blocker

Available as: 25 mg, 50 mg, and 100 mg tablets; 5 mg/ml solution for injection

metoprolol succinate

Brand name: *Toprol-XL*

Classification: beta-1 adrenergic blocker

Available as: 50 mg, 100 mg, and 200 mg extended-release tablets

metoprolol tartrate

Brand name: *Lopressor*

Classification: beta-1 adrenergic blocker

Available as: 50 mg and 100 mg tablets; 1 mg/ml solution for injection

doxazocin mesylate

Brand name: *Cardura*

Classification: alpha adrenergic receptor antagonist

Available as: 1 mg, 2 mg, 4 mg, and 8 mg tablets

prazocin hydrochloride

Brand name: *Minipress*

Classification: alpha-1 adrenergic receptor antagonist

Available as: 1 mg, 2 mg, and 5 mg capsules

clonidine hydrochloride

Brand name: *Catapres*

Classification: centrally acting sympathoplegic

Available as: 0.1 mg, 0.2 mg, and 0.3 mg tablets; transdermal patch releasing 0.1 mg, 0.2 mg, or 0.3 mg/hr

methyldopa

Brand name: *Aldomet*

Classification: centrally acting sympathoplegic

Available as: 125 mg, 250 mg, and 500 mg tablets; 250 mg/5 ml oral suspension; 250 mg/5 ml solution for injection

hydralazine hydrochloride

Brand name: *Apresoline*

Classification: peripheral vasodilator

Available as: 10 mg, 25 mg, 50 mg, and 100 mg tablets; 20 mg/ml solution for injection

benazepril hydrochloride

Brand name: *Lotensin*

Classification: angiotensin converting enzyme (ACE) inhibitor

Available as: 5 mg, 10 mg, 20 mg, and 40 mg tablets

captopril

Brand name: *Capoten*

Classification: ACE inhibitor

Available as: 12.5 mg, 25 mg, 50 mg, and 100 mg tablets

enalapril

Brand name: *Vasotec*

Classification: ACE inhibitor

Available as: 2.5 mg, 5 mg, 10 mg, and 20 mg tablets; 1.25 mg/ml solution for injection

fosinopril

Brand name: *Monopril*

Classification: ACE inhibitor

Available as: 10 mg, 20 mg, and 40 mg tablets

lisinopril

Brand names: *Prinivil, Zestril*

Classification: ACE inhibitor

Available as: 2.5 mg, 5 mg, 10 mg, 20 mg, and 40 mg tablets

enalapril maleate with hydrochlorothiazide

Brand name: *Vaseretic*

Classification: combination drug — ACE inhibitor with diuretic

Available as: 5 mg enalapril + 12.5 mg thiazide, and 10 mg enalapril + 25 mg thiazide tablets

losartan potassium

Brand name: *Cozaar*

Classification: angiotensin II receptor blocker

Available as: 25 mg and 50 mg tablets

Drugs Used for Angina Pectoris

nitroglycerin sublingual

Major brand name: *Nitrostat*

Classification: coronary vasodilator

Available as: 0.3 mg, 0.4 mg, and 0.6 mg tablets; sublingual spray and patch

verapamil hydrochloride

Major brand names: *Calan, Isoptin, Verelan*

Classification: calcium channel blocker

Available as: 2.5 mg/ml solution for injection; 120 mg, 180 mg, 240 mg, and 360 mg extended-release capsules; 40 mg, 80 mg, and 120 mg extended-release tablets

Drugs Dispensed for Congestive Heart Failure

digoxin

Brand names: *Lanoxicaps, Lanoxin*

Classification: cardiac glycoside

Available as: 0.05 mg, 0.1 mg, and 0.2 mg capsules; 0.125 mg, 0.25 mg, and 0.5 mg tablets; 0.05 mg/ml elixir; 0.1 mg/ml and 0.25 mg/ml injection

Drugs Used in the Therapy of Arrythmias

disopyramide

Brand name: *Norpace*

Classification: Class I sodium channel blocker

Available as: 100 mg and 150 mg capsules

lidocaine hydrochloride

Brand name: *Xylocaine*

Classification: Class II sodium channel blocker, antiarrythmic

Available as: 10 mg/ml, 20 mg/ml, 40 mg/ml, 100 mg/ml, and 200 mg/ml solution for injection; premixed IV solution

Drugs Used to Reduce Cholesterol

fluvastatin sodium

Brand name: *Lescol*

Classification: enzyme inhibitor (HMG-CoA reductase)

Available as: 20 mg and 40 mg capsules

gemfibrozil

Brand name: *Lopid*

Classification: inhibitor of triglyceride formation

Available as: 600 mg tablet

lovastatin (mevinolin)

Brand name: *Mevacor*

Classification: enzyme inhibitor (HMG-CoA reductase)

Available as: 10 mg, 20 mg, and 40 mg tablets

simvastatin

Brand name: *Zocor*

Classification: enzyme inhibitor (HMG-CoA reductase)

Available as: 5 mg, 10 mg, 20 mg, and 40 mg tablets

Drugs That Decrease Clotting

ticlopidine hydrochloride

Brand name: *Ticlid*

Classification: antithrombotic

Available as: 250 mg tablet

warfarin sodium

Brand name: *Coumadin*

Classification: anticoagulant — inhibitor of vitamin K recycling

Available as: 1 mg, 2 mg, 2.5 mg, 4 mg, 5 mg, 7.5 mg, and 10 mg tablets; 5 mg powder for injection

Drugs That Decrease Blood Viscosity

pentoxifylline

Brand name: *Trental*

Classification/use: drug that increases tissue perfusion

Available as: 400 mg extended-release tablet

Drugs for Decreasing Fluid Volume (Diuretics)

acetazolamide

Brand name: *Diamox*

Classification: carbonic anhydrase inhibitor

Available as: 125 mg and 250 mg tablets; 500 mg sustained-release tablet; 500 mg powder for injection; opthalmic solution

amiloride hydrochloride

Brand name: *Midamor*

Classification: potassium-sparing diuretic

Available as: 5 mg tablet

spironolactone

Brand name: *Aldactone*

Classification: inhibitor of aldosterone, potassium-sparing diuretic

Available as: 20 mg, 50 mg, and 100 mg tablets

bumetanide

Brand name: *Bumex*

Classification: loop diuretic

Available as: 0.5 mg, 1 mg, and 2 mg tablets; 0.5 mg/2 ml solution for injection

furosemide

Major brand names: *Lasix*, *Myrosemide*

Classification: loop diuretic

Available as: 20 mg, 40 mg, and 80 mg tablets; 10 mg/ml solution for injection

hydrochlorothiazide

Major brand names: *Esidrex*, *Ezide*, *Oretic*

Classification: thiazide diuretic

Available as: 12.5 mg capsules; 25 mg, 50 mg, and 100 mg tablets; 50 mg/5 ml oral solution

triamterine and hydrochlorothiazide

Brand names: *Dyazide, Maxzide*

Classification: combination drug, diuretic

Available as: 25 mg thiazide/50 mg triamterine, and 50 mg thiazide/100 mg triamterine capsules; 25 mg thiazide/37.5 mg triamterine, and 50 mg thiazide/75 mg triamterine tablets

demeclocycline hydrochloride

Brand name: *Declomycin*

Classification: antidiuretic hormone (ADH) antagonist; this drug is an antibiotic which also antagonizes ADH and is used primarily in the therapy of inappropriate ADH secretion.

Available as: 150 mg and 300 mg tablets; 300 mg capsule

Drugs That Increase Pulmonary Ventilation

Steroid Drugs

beclomethasone dipropionate

Brand names: *Beclovent, Vanceril, Vanceril DS*

Classification: glucocorticoid

Available as: 0.42 mg/dose metered dose inhaler; 0.42 mg/dose and 0.84 mg/dose nasal spray

fluticasone propionate

Major brand names: *Flonase, Flovent*

Classification: glucocorticoid

Available as: 0.11 mg/dose, 0.22 mg/dose, and 0.44 mg/dose metered dose inhaler; 0.05 mg/dose nasal spray; 0.005% ointment; 0.05% cream

methylprednisolone

Brand name: *Medrol*

Classification: corticosteriod, anti-inflammatory

Available as: 2 mg, 4 mg, 8 mg, 16 mg, 24 mg, and 32 mg tablets; 12 mg/ml, 40 mg/ml, and 80 mg/ml solution for injection (acetate form); 40 mg, 125 mg, 500 mg, 1 g, and 2 g powder for injection (sodium succinate form)

prednisone

Brand names: *Deltazone, Meticorten, Panasol-S, Orasone 1, 5, 10, 20, and 50*

Classification: corticosteroid, anti-inflammatory

Available as: 1 mg, 2.5 mg, 5 mg, 10 mg, 20 mg, and 50 mg tablets; 5 mg/ml concentrate; 5 mg/5 ml solution; 5 mg/5 ml syrup

Drugs That Affect the Sympathetic Nervous System

albuterol

Major brand names: *Proventil, Ventolin*

Classification: beta adrenergic agonist

Available as: 0.09 mg/dose metered dose inhaler; 0.083% and 0.5% solution; 2 mg/5 ml syrup; 200 mcg capsule; 2 mg and 4 mg tablet; 4 mg and 8 mg extended-release tablets.

ipratropium bromide

Brand name: *Atrovent*

Classification: cholinergic antagonist, quaternary ammonium

Available as: 0.018 mg/dose metered dose inhaler; 0.03% nasal spray; 0.02% solution for inhalation

salmeterol xinafoate

Brand name: *Serevent*

Classification: beta-2 adrenergic agonist

Available as: 21 mcg/dose inhaler

Drugs Used to Relieve Allergies (Antihistamines)

fexofenadine hydrochloride

Brand name: *Allegra*

Classification: Antihistamine, piperidine type

Available as: 60 mg capsule

loratidine

Brand name: *Claritin*

Classification: antihistamine

Available as: 10 mg tablet; 5 mg/5 ml syrup

Drugs That Affect the Gastrointestinal System

Drugs That Decrease the Secretion of Stomach Acid — Histamine (H₂) Receptor Antagonists

cimetidine hydrochloride

Brand name: *Tagamet*

Available as: 100 mg, 200 mg, 300 mg, 400 mg, and 800 mg tablets; 150 mg/ml and 300 mg/50 ml solution for injection

famotidine

Brand name: *Pepcid*

Available as: 10 mg, 20 mg, and 40 mg tablets; 10 mg/ml solution for injection; 40 mg/5 ml powder for reconstitution

nizatidine

Brand name: *Axid*

Available as: 75 mg tablet; 150 mg and 300 mg capsule

ranitidine hydrochloride

Brand name: *Zantac*

Available as: 75 mg, 150 mg, and 300 mg tablets; 150 mg effervescent tablet; 150 mg and 300 mg capsules; 150 mg granules for reconstitution; 15 mg/ml syrup; 1 mg/ml and 25 mg/ml injection

Drugs That Decrease Stomach Acid Synthesis

omeprazole

Brand name: *Prilosec*

Available as: 10 mg and 20 mg enteric coated capsules

Drugs Used to Prevent Ulcers

misoprostol

Brand name: *Cytotec*

Classification: synthetic prostaglandin, antiulcer drug

Available as: 100 mcg and 200 mcg tablets

Drugs for Use in Parasitic Infections

mebendazole

Brand name: *Vermox*

Classification: anthelmintic, metabolic enzyme inhibitor

Available as: 100 mg chewable tablets

thiabendazole

Brand name: *Mintezol*

Classification: anthelmintic, metabolic enzyme inhibitor

Available as: 500 mg chewable tablets; 500 mg/5 ml suspension

Drugs That Affect the Endocrine System

Drugs Used to Control Diabetes Mellitus

Type I diabetes (insulin dependent)

human NPH insulin (isophane)

Brand names: *Humulin, Novolin*

Classification: human insulin, intermediate acting

Available as: 100 U/ml insulin for subcutaneous injection

porcine (pork) NPH insulin (isophane)

Brand names: *NPH-N, NPH Iletin II*

Classification: porcine insulin, intermediate acting

Available as: 100 U/ml insulin for subcutaneous injection

bovine (beef) NPH insulin

Brand name: *Beef NPH insulin*

Classification: bovine insulin, intermediate acting

Available as: 100 U/ml insulin for injection

combination beef/pork NPH insulin

Brand name: *NPH Iletin*

Classification: beef/pork insulin, intermediate acting

Available as: 100 U/ml insulin for subcutaneous injection

Type II diabetes (non-insulin dependent)

glipizide

Brand names: *Glucotrol, Glucotrol XL*

Classification: oral sulfonylurea antidiabetic

Available as: 5 mg and 10 mg tablets; 5 mg and 10 mg extended-release tablets

glyburide

Brand names: *DiaBeta, Micronase*

Classification: oral sulfonylurea antidiabetic

Available as: 1.25 mg, 1.5 mg, 2.5 mg, 3 mg, 5 mg, and 6 mg tablets

metformin hydrochloride

Brand name: *Glucophage*

Classification: biguanide-type antihyperglycemic drug

Available as: 500 mg and 850 mg tablets

Drugs for Therapy of Hypothyroidism

levothyroxine

Brand names: *Synthroid, Levothroid, Eltroxin*

Classification: thyroid hormone replacement

Available as: 0.2 mg and 0.5 mg powder for injection; 0.025 mg, 0.05 mg, 0.075 mg, 0.088 mg, 0.1 mg, 0.112 mg, 0.125 mg, 0.137 mg, 0.15 mg, 0.175 mg, 0.2 mg, 0.3 mg, and 0.5 mg tablets

(Dosages less than 1 mg are normally expressed in mcg, e.g., 25 mcg)

Drugs That Affect the Reproductive System

Estrogens

Note: All estrogenic drugs must be dispensed with a mandatory package insert for the patient.

conjugated estrogens

Brand name: *Premarin*

Classification: estrogen, natural

Available as: 0.3 mg, 0.625 mg, 0.9 mg, 1.25 mg, and 2.5 mg tablets; 25 mg/ml powder for injection; 0.625 mg/g vaginal cream

estradiol

Brand name: *Estrace*

Available as: 0.5 mg, 1 mg, 2 mg tablets; 0.1 mg.g cream

dienestrol

Brand name: *OrthoDienestrol*

Available as: 10 mg/g cream

estropipate

Brand name: *Ogen*

Available as: 0.625 mg, 1.25 mg, 2.5 mg tablets; 1.5 mg/g cream

quinestrol

Brand name: *Estrovis*

Available as: 100 mcg tablet

Estrogen Antagonists (Anti-Estrogens)

anastrozole

Brand name: *Arimidex*

Available as: 1 mg tablet

clomiphene

Brand names: *Clomid, Serophene, Milophene*

Available as: 50 mg tablet

finasteride

Brand name: *Proscar*

Available as: 5 mg tablet

tamoxifen citrate

Brand name: *Nolvadex*

Classification: competitive antagonist of estradiol

Available as: 10 mg and 20 mg tablets

Progestins

hydroxyprogesterone caproate

Brand name: *Delalutin*

Classification: competitive antagonist of estradiol

Available as: 125 mg/ml and 250 mg/ml solution for intramuscular injection

medroxyprogesterone acetate

Brand names: *Amen, Cycrin, Depo-Provera, Provera*

Available as: 2.5 mg, 5 mg, and 10 mg tablets; 150 mg/ml and 400 mg/ml solution for injection

norethindrone

Brand names: *Norlutin, Micronol, Nor - Q.D.*

Available as: 5 mg tablet (Norlutin), 0.35 mg tablet (Micronol, Nor - Q.D.)

norgestrel

Brand names: *Ovrette*

Available as: 75 mcg tablet

Androgens

fluoxymestrone

Brand name: *Halotestin*

Available as: 2 mg, 5 mg, and 10 mg tablets

oxandrolone

Brand names: *Oxandrin*

Available as: 2.5 mg tablet

Drugs Used for Infection

Penicillin and Derivatives

amoxicillin (amoxycillin)

Major brand names: *Amoxil, Polymox*

Classification: bactericidal antibiotic

Available as: 250 mg and 500 mg capsules; 125 mg and 250 mg chewable tablets; 50 mg/ml, 125 mg/5 ml, and 250 mg/5 ml powder for reconstitution

oral penicillin

Major brand names: *Pen-Vee K, BeepenVK*

Classification: bactericidal antibiotic, inhibitor of bacterial cell wall formation

Available as: 250 mg and 500 mg tablets; 124 mg/ml and 250 mg/ml powder for reconstitution

loracarbef

Brand name: *Lorabid*

Classification: Beta-lactam antibiotic

Available as: 200 mg and 400 mg capsules; 100 mg/5 ml and 200 mg/5 ml powder for reconstitution

Cephalosporin Antibiotics

cephalexin hydrochloride monohydrate

Brand name: Keftab

Available as: 500 mg tablet

cephalexin monohydrate

Brand names: *Biocef, Keflex*

Available as: 250 mg and 500 mg capsules; 250 mg and 500 mg tablets; 125 mg/5 ml and 250 mg/5 ml powder for reconstitution

cefaclor

Brand name: *Ceclor*

Available as: 250 mg and 500 mg capsules

Macrolide antibiotics

erythromycin base

Major brand names: *E-Mycin, Ery-Tab, Robimycin Robitabs, Aknemycin, Staticin, Theramycin Z, T-Stat*

Classification: bacteriostatic antibiotic, inhibitor of bacterial protein synthesis

Available as: 250 mg enteric coated capsule; 250 mg and 500 mg tablets; 333 mg and 500 mg tablets/coated particles; 250 mg, 333 mg, and 500 mg enteric coated tablets. 2% gel/jelly; 2% ointment; 5 mg/g ophthalmic ointment; 2% pad; 1.5% and 2% solution; 2% swab

erythromycin stearate

Brand name: *Eramycin*

Classification: bacteriostatic antibiotic, inhibitor of bacterial protein synthesis

Available: 250 mg and 500 mg tablets

azithromycin dihydrate

Brand name: *Zithromax*

Classification: bacteriostatic antibiotic, bacterial ribosomal function inhibitor

Available as: 250 mg capsule; 600 mg tablet; 100 mg/5 ml, 200 mg/5 ml, and 1 g/packet powder for reconstitution

clarithromycin

Brand name: *Biaxin*

Classification: macrolide antibiotic, bacterial protein synthesis inhibitor

Available as: 250 mg and 500 mg tablets; 125 mg/5 ml and 250 mg/5 ml granules for reconstitution

nitrofurantoin

Major brand names: *Macrodantin, Macrobid*

Classification: macrolide antibiotic, bacteriostatic, inhibitor of bacterial protein synthesis

Available: 25 mg, 50 mg, and 100 mg capsules; 25 mg/5 ml suspension

Fluoroquinolone Antibiotics

ciprofloxacin

Brand names: *Cipro*

Classification: DNA topoisomerase (Types II and IV) inhibitor

Available as: 250 mg and 500 mg tablets; cystitis pack; solution for injection; ophthalmic solution

ofloxacin

Brand names: *Floxin, Ocuflox*

Classification: DNA topoisomerase (Types II and IV) inhibitor

Available as: 200 mg, 300 mg, and 400 mg tablets; 0.3% ophthalmic solution; 4 mg/ml, 20 mg/ml, and 40 mg/ml solution for injection

Tetracycline Antibiotics

tetracycline hydrochloride

Major brand names: *Achromycin V, Nor-Tet, Sumycin*

Classification: bacteriostatic antibiotic, inhibitor of bacterial protein synthesis

Available as: 250 mg and 500 mg tablets; 100 mg, 250 mg, and 500 mg capsules; 2.2 mg/ml oral solution; 125 mg/5 ml syrup; 3% ointment; 1% ophthalmic solution

Combination Drugs

trimethoprim/sulfamethoxazole

Major brand names: *Bactrim, Cotrim, Septra*

Classification: combination of antimetabolite antibiotic and sulfa antibiotic

Available as: 80 mg trimethoprim/400 sulfamethoxazole tablets; 160 mg trimethoprim/800 mg sulfamethoxazole double strength tablets; 40 mg trimethoprim and 200 mg sulfamethoxazole /5 ml oral suspension; 16 mg trimethoprim and 80 mg sulfamethoxazole /ml concentrate for injection

Antiviral Drugs

acyclovir

Brand name: *Zovirax*

Available as: 200 mg capsule; 400 mg and 800 mg tablets; 500 mg and 1000 mg powder for injection; 200 mg/5 ml suspension; 5% ointment

Antifungal Drugs

fluconazole

Brand name: *Diflucan*

Classification: antifungal, enzyme inhibitor (fungal cytochrome P450)

Available as: 50 mg, 100 mg, 150 mg, and 200 mg tablets; 50 mg/5 ml and 200 mg/5 ml powder for reconstitution; 2 mg/ml, 200 mg/100 ml, and 400 mg/200 ml solution for injection

ketoconazole

Brand name: *Nizoral*

Classification: fungal cell membrane synthesis inhibitor

Available as: 2% cream; 2% shampoo; 200 mg tablet

Questions for Review

1. A drug used for hypertension that would affect the vascular system is:
   1. Norvasc.
   2. Timoptic.
   3. Diamox.
   4. Cefobid.

2. Which of the following are antibiotics?
   1. Keflex
   2. Ceclor
   3. Polymox
   4. All of the above
   5. 1 and 2 only

3. Which of the following is a diuretic?
   1. Haldol
   2. Lasix
   3. Thorazine
   4. Both 1 and 2

4. Which of the following is not used for treating depression?
   1. Elavil
   2. Prozac
   3. Paxil
   4. None of the above

5. Which of the following directly affect(s) the cardiovascular system?
   1. Cardizem
   2. Cardura
   3. Catapres
   4. All of the above
   5. 1 and 2

6. Which of the following is an antifungal drug?
   1. miconazole
   2. cefamandole
   3. Tegopen
   4. Hydrocort

7. Which of the following is not a penicillin drug?
   1. Geocillin
   2. Geopen
   3. pentoxifylline
   4. Beepen-K

8. Which of the following might be a long-lasting form of nitroglycerine?
    1. Nitro-bid
    2. Nitrostat
    3. Nitro-dur
    4. Nitropress

9. Which of the drugs in Problem 8 is not a form of nitrogylcerine at all?

Solutions to Questions for Review

The purpose of this exercise is to see if you can determine what the drug does from the name. (This may not always be possible; some names simply must be memorized.)

1. If a drug affects the vascular system, it may have a derivation of a word for vessel in the name, such as *vaso* or *vasc*. The correct answer is **1**. Norvasc is a calcium channel blocker (amlodipine).

2. *Keflex* and *Ceclor* are *cephalosporin* antibiotics, and *Polymox* is *amoxicillin*. The correct answer is **4**.

3. This one is harder. *Lasix* is the only diuretic (named because it *lasts six* hours). The correct answer is **2**.

4. All of these drugs are antidepressants. The correct answer is **4**.

5. Drugs that affect the cardiovascular system often have some form of *cardio* in the name, much like the ones that affect the vessels have vaso. *Cardizem*, a calcium channel blocker, would affect both the heart and the vessels, while *Cardura*, an alpha receptor blocker, would affect the vessels and speed up the heart by reflex action. The correct answer is **5**.

6. Antifungal drugs (generic names) often end in ole. The only possible answers are 1 and 2. However, cefamandole (#2) begins with cef, so it is a good bet it's a cephalosporin antibiotic. The correct answer is **1**.

7. This is a good example of look-alike and sound-alike drugs. Three of these names contain *pen*, and one contains *cillin*. Of the *pen* drugs, the only one with the *pen* in the beginning of the name is pentoxifylline. The drug is actually a blood thinner. The correct answer is **3**.

8. Here, we are looking for something that says "long lasting." All of them start with *Nitro*, but the only one that ends in *dur* (like in *durable*) is Nitro-Dur. The correct answer is **3**.

9. This one requires memorization, although the generic and brand names sound very much alike. Nitropress is nitroprusside. The correct answer is **4**.

Chapter 27

The Pharmacology of Drug Interactions

Quick Study

(See text for full explanation.)

I. **General mechanisms of drug interactions**

   A. Absorption

   B. Distribution

   C. Clearance

   D. Drug mechanism

     • *Synergism:* therapeutic and toxic effects

     • *Additive effects*

     • *Antagonism*

Ways In Which Drugs Can Interact

There are many ways in which drugs can interact with each other within the body to cause problems. Many adverse interactions happen because the drugs do different things that interfere with their **mechanism**, or the way that they work. Many others occur because of the way that the drugs are stored or distributed within the body or the way in which they are eliminated from the body. The following interactions are described: absorption, distribution, and protein binding.

Absorption

In order for a drug to work, it must be *free* and *in the bloodstream*. Thus, if it is taken orally, the drug must be *absorbed* from the gastrointestinal (GI) tract into the bloodstream. Sometimes, two drugs are absorbed into the body in the same way and so interfere with each other's absorption by competing for transport sites into the body.

In the same way, some drugs decrease the absorption of other drugs by binding to them in the stomach or intestine and preventing their absorption into the body. For example, sucralfate, a drug used to promote healing of the stomach lining, binds to many drugs in the digestive tract and prevents or decreases their absorption; the tetracycline drugs (tetracycline, doxycycline, minocycline, etc.), if taken with meals or with mineral supplements (which contain iron, calcium, and magnesium), bind to these minerals in the intestine and cannot be absorbed into the body.

The acidity or alkalinity (pH) of two drugs taken together can influence the absorption of a drug as well. For example, antacids or histamine blockers (cimetidine, ranitidine), which decrease stomach acidity, will decrease the amount of aspirin or other acidic drugs absorbed into the body, thus decreasing the drug's effectiveness. (Acidic drugs are absorbed well in the acid environment of the stomach. Antacids decrease the acidity of the stomach and thus decrease the absorption of acidic drugs.) Changes in body pH due to the ingestion of an acidic or alkaline drug or substance can influence the rate of clearance of the drug as well (see below).

Absorption of a drug is also influenced by the route of administration. Drugs injected intramuscularly are absorbed more slowly than drugs injected intravenously (which are technically not absorbed at all since the drug goes directly into the bloodstream). Including a vasoconstrictor, or local anesthetic, such as procaine, will reduce the rate of absorption even further, allowing more drug to be injected with a slower absorption rate ("long-acting" formulations).

Drug Distribution

Once the drug is in the bloodstream, it disseminates throughout the body, or is **distributed**. Part of the drug will be free in the plasma (this is the drug that will actually be working in the body). The rest may be stored in some way, such as bound to plasma proteins, or stored in fat. Binding of the drug to plasma proteins stabilizes the drug and also keeps it from being broken down by the liver or filtered out and excreted by the kidneys (the proteins are too big to be filtered out). Remember that a drug, in order to work, must be free in the plasma—a stored drug is not available to work. The more free drug in the plasma, the greater is the effect and there is greater potential for toxicity.

Protein Binding Interactions

Many drug interactions occur because two or more drugs bind to the same plasma proteins. The one that binds the tightest and the fastest "wins," leaving the "loser" floating in the plasma. This results in too much of the "loser" drug as free drug in the plasma. Since free drug is available to work in the body, this drug may cause toxic effects. In addition, because the free drug is more quickly metabolized or filtered out by the kidney, this drug will be eliminated from the body faster, as well. When two drugs that both bind extensively to plasma proteins are taken concurrently, the doses must be adjusted to reflect the change in plasma free drug concentrations.

An example of a drug that is highly protein bound is warfarin (Coumadin). This drug has protein-binding interactions with many drugs.

Drug Clearance

Whenever a patient takes a drug, that drug is designed to do its job and leave. The body eliminates the drug after a period of time by breaking it down with enzymes (metabolism) in the liver and/or using the kidneys to filter it out of the blood and dump it in the urine. Drugs that are metabolized may go into the bile and out through the intestine, or, if the actions of the enzymes in the liver make them water soluble (so that they can be dissolved easily in water), they may go out through the urine. Some drugs are not metabolized; if they are soluble enough in water, they may go directly out in the urine.

A very important drug interaction occurs when more than one drug is being metabolized at the same time (this includes drugs such as alcohol). Some drugs interact by competing with each other for the same enzyme or altering the activity of a liver enzyme. Enzymes are proteins that break down drugs. Many drugs are metabolized by a particular group of enzymes called cytochrome P450. Drugs such as cimetidine (Tagamet) alter the activity and amount of these enzymes, which decreases the metabolism of other drugs that use it. This means that the drug levels in the blood will increase as the patient keeps taking the prescribed doses.

An important thing to consider is a patient's age. Because drugs are cleared out of the body by the liver and kidney and the functions of these organs decrease with age, the dosage of the drug must be adjusted to compensate. Another important factor, especially when assessing drugs eliminated by the liver, is whether the patient is an abuser of alcohol or has preexisting liver damage (e.g., from hepatitis). Any existing damage to the liver could decrease the rate of clearance of the drug, causing the blood levels of drug to build up to toxic levels over time.

Drug Toxicity and Interactions

All drugs are, to some extent, poisons and have harmful effects. The dosages established for the patient are designed to minimize the harmful effects while maximizing the beneficial effects. However, taking more than one drug concurrently may cause a problem; sometimes one drug can set the stage for the harmful effects (toxic effects) of another. For instance, drugs like isoproterenol (a sympathetic agonist at beta receptors) act on the heart to increase heart rate and increase electrical conduction through the heart tissue. Too much can cause tachycardia and arrythmias. Thyroid drugs sensitize the heart to the effects of norepinephrine and epinephrine which are produced under stress (and have effects on the heart similar to isoproterenol). Taking thyroid hormone (or just being hyperthyroid) while taking a drug like isoproterenol could increase the sensitivity of the heart to the toxic effects of the drug and result in severe arrythmias.

Drugs like furosemide and thiazide diuretics cause a large amount of potassium excretion. The heart is very sensitive to potassium, and particularly when other drugs which alter potassium levels are taken concurrently (e.g., digitalis glycosides), the loss of potassium can lead to severe arrythmias.

Additive, Synergistic, and Antagonistic Effects

Drugs that produce the same physiological effects may behave differently when taken together. For example, if two drugs both lower blood pressure by the same mechanism (e.g., blocking calcium channels) and both are seen to lower systolic pressure by 5%, then, by taking both drugs concurrently, we would expect a 10% decrease in systolic pressure. This is called an *additive* effect - the amount of effect of one drug is adding to that of another. If instead these two drugs did not work by the same mechanism—say, one drug blocked calcium channels, reducing systolic pressure by 5%, and the other blocked norepinephrine receptors (also reducing systolic pressure by 5%)—taking both drugs concurrently might produce a decrease of *15%*. This is called *synergism*—two drugs taken together producing a physiological effect which is much greater than the effects of each drug added together (5% + 5% = 10%, not 15%). In contrast, a drug may *interfere* with the actions of another, reducing the physiological effect. This is called *antagonism*.

Some drugs produce similar *toxic* effects and should not be used together. For example, furosemide and streptomycin both produce ototoxicity—furosemide lowers the fluid volume in the inner ear reducing stimulation of the auditory nerve, and aminoglycoside antibiotics, such as streptomycin, are directly toxic to the auditory nerve. When these drugs are taken alone, the effects are manageable; however, when taken concurrently the effect on the auditory nerve more than doubles. These drugs synergize to produce a very large detrimental effect on the ear, with much more ototoxicity than would be expected.

Another common example is the interaction between a central nervous system (CNS) depressant and an antihistamine. Antihistamines produce a small amount of CNS depression, some more than others. However, when antihistamines are taken with another drug that produces CNS depression, such as anticonvulsants or antipsychotics, the effect can be lethal. The same is true with ethyl alcohol, which is an extremely potent CNS depressant. If alcoholic beverages are taken with drugs such as antiseizure medications, antipsychotics, antidepressants, and similar drugs that produce CNS depression (particularly barbiturates, which can be lethal by themselves, if abused), the central and autonomic nervous systems can be depressed to an extent that they are unable to function, and death could result. Since the depressant effect is so much greater when both drugs are taken concurrently, this is a **synergistic** reaction.

Some drugs may synergize to produce too much of a beneficial effect, for example, aspirin and warfarin. Aspirin is an **antithrombotic** drug; it affects platelets in the blood, to make them less "sticky," reducing the formation of small **thrombi** (clots). The reduction in the "stickiness" of the platelets may decrease the activity of clotting factors on the platelets, as well, and thus reduce clotting. Warfarin is an **anticoagulant** that works by interfering with the recycling of vitamin K, which is required for many of these clotting factors to work properly. When aspirin and warfarin are taken together, the effects of the two drugs synergize and blood clotting is decreased to the extent that internal bleeding may occur.

In contrast, the antithrombotic drugs aspirin and dipyridamole are an example of drugs which have additive effects. Since both drugs have the same physiological effect (inhibition of platelet function), the overall effect of combination therapy will be predictable—approximately the sum of the effects from each drug. Concurrent therapy may be beneficial, as lower doses of each drug may be given, reducing the level of side effects from each drug, while the therapeutic effect is maintained.

Some drugs may **antagonize** (block) the effects of others. For example, a blood pressure medication such as propranolol, which blocks adrenergic beta receptors, should not be taken concurrently with a decongestant, such as phenylpropanolamine (also used as a diet aid) or an amphetamine, because drugs such as these increase the amount of norepinephrine in the system, which results in increased stimulation of adrenergic receptors. A monoamine oxidase inhibitor, such as tranylcypromine (Parnate), used for depression, would also raise levels of norepinephrine (and epinephrine) by inhibiting its breakdown. This would antagonize the effects of a drug such as propranolol which is designed to *block* the effects of norepinephrine.

In addition to interactions between *drugs* in the body, there are also many drugs which interact with chemicals found in certain foods that should be avoided during therapy. It is the responsibility of the pharmacy as well as the prescriber to be sure that the patient knows to avoid these types of foods. For example, the anticoagulant warfarin has a drug-food interaction. As discussed previously, warfarin (Coumadin) inhibits the recycling of vitamin K by the liver, which decreases the activity of the vitamin K dependent clotting factors. Vitamin K is present in foods such as green leafy vegetables. These types of foods should be avoided during therapy, as vitamin K absorbed from the vegetables replaces vitamin K lost through the action of the drug, and reduces the efficacy of the drug (a drug-food antagonism).

Another drug-food interaction involves MAO inhibitors. These drugs inhibit the breakdown of norepinephrine. A chemical called tyramine is present in foods such as cheese, chocolate, wine, and other types of food and drink. Tyramine causes norepinephrine to be released in large quantities. If these foods are eaten during therapy, large amounts of norepinephrine will be produced which now cannot be broken down, as breakdown of norepinephrine has been inhibited by the drug. The rapid increase in norepinephrine levels can cause a hypertensive crisis which could be fatal (a drug-food synergism).

Drugs That Affect the Autonomic Nervous System

Drugs that alter the effects of the autonomic nervous system (ANS) are probably among the most frequently dispensed drugs. Discharge of the sympathetic nervous system in the body (release of norepinephrine or epinephrine) causes vasoconstriction and increases the levels of angiotensin II (both of which increase blood pressure), increases heart rate and force of contraction (also contributing to increased blood pressure), and releases stored energy (causing an increase in blood sugar). Many of the drugs that are marketed for hypertension interfere with the action of the sympathetic nervous system. As **antagonists**, these drugs block the receptors on the cells which allow the norepinephrine (and epinephrine) to act. When the effects of the sympathetic system are blocked, the effects of the **parasympathetic** system are seen: the heart slows down and vessels dilate, thus decreasing blood pressure.

Therapeutic Manipulation of the Sympathetic Nervous System

We can get specific therapeutic effects by blocking or stimulating specific receptors for norepinephrine and epinephrine. Beta$_1$ receptor blocking drugs such as propranolol or atenolol slow down the heart directly, lowering cardiac output and blood pressure. Alpha$_1$ receptor blocking agents, such as phentolamine and doxazocin, inhibit vasoconstriction, which results in a dilation of arterioles and lowering of systemic blood pressure (hint: drugs such as propranolol and phentolamine would have synergistic effects). Drugs which affect the alpha$_2$ receptor, however, would have effects which might seem opposite—drugs such as clonidine, an alpha$_2$ receptor *agonist*, would decrease the release of norepinephrine and thus decrease sympathetic effects all together, resulting in a decrease in systemic blood pressure. Note that drugs which stimulate a particular receptor (agonists) and those which block the receptor (antagonists) should not be prescribed at the same time, even for different therapeutic reasons.

A **cholinergic blocking agent** such as atropine also causes an increase in sympathetic effects, as the parasympathetic effects are blocked. It is important to remember, when thinking about drugs that affect the autonomic nervous system, that both the parasympathetic and sympathetic effects are always present in every organ in the body. One of them is just the "strongest." Which one is dominant depends on factors like stress, emotion, and degree of activity. If the effects of one are blocked, the effects of the other will be seen. So if a patient is taking a drug that blocks sympathetic effects, parasympathetic effects are seen, and vice-versa.

Medical contraindications of drugs which affect the sympathetic nervous system

It is also important to remember that drugs interact with physical conditions as well as with other drugs. The most common of these are cardiovascular disease and diabetes. If a person with diabetes takes a drug such as isoproterenol (or even phenylpropanolamine, a decongestant), the drug will cause fats to be broken down (a sympathetic nervous system action) and blood sugar to rise, which diabetics cannot handle due to a lack of insulin. Those with cardiovascular disease may not be able to tolerate antihypertensive drugs that decrease contraction of the heart (e.g., verapamil), because the heart may already be enlarged and not contracting properly. There are many factors to be considered that are beyond the scope of this text.

Questions for Review

1. Which of the following drugs have a major drug-drug interaction?
    1. Isoproterenol and furosemide
    2. Digitalis and mannitol
    3. Secobarbital and alcohol
    4. Aspirin and diazepam

2. The action or potency of which of the following would be affected by concurrent use of antacids, such as calcium carbonate (Tums)?
   1. Aspirin
   2. Ibuprofen
   3. Doxycycline
   4. Cimetidine
   5. Both 1 and 3

3. Which of the following would not have a synergistic action?
   1. Warfarin and aspirin
   2. Haloperidol and diphenhydramine
   3. Furosemide and verapamil
   4. Sodium valproate and alcohol

4. The dose of which of the following might have to be adjusted in the elderly?
   1. Drugs that are excreted through the bile
   2. Drugs that are stored in body fat
   3. Drugs that cross into the brain
   4. Drugs that are excreted only by the kidneys

5. Which of the following may affect platelets?
   1. Coumadin
   2. Aspirin
   3. Heparin
   4. Inderal

6. Drugs such as isoproterenol might be contraindicated in which types of patients?
   1. Elderly
   2. Diabetics
   3. Those with renal insufficiency
   4. Women prone to miscarriages

7. Drugs that are stored bound to plasma proteins in the blood, such as Tegretol, would interact most with
   1. heparin.
   2. thyroid hormone.
   3. warfarin.
   4. cimetidine.

Solutions to Questions for Review

1. The synergistic sedation produced by the barbiturate and the alcohol would make #3 the best answer. The correct answer is **3.**

2. The change in pH of the stomach due to less acid would change the absorption of aspirin. Also, because there is a divalent ion present (calcium) in the antacid, tetracycline-type drugs would be complexed in the intestine and would not be absorbed. The correct answer is **5.**

3. Both warfarin and aspirin would seriously affect clotting. Haloperidol (an antipsychotic) and diphenhydramine (an antihistamine) would both cause CNS depression and would synergize, as would the sodium valproate/alcohol combination. The correct answer is **3.**

4. Both renal clearance and hepatic clearance decline in the elderly, but renal function is the biggest issue. The correct answer is **4.**

5. Only aspirin directly affects platelets. The correct answer is **2.**

6. Drugs such as isoproterenol increase the rate and force of contraction of the heart. Also, because they stimulate beta receptors, they increase blood sugar. The correct answer is **2.**

7. The interaction here would be a competition between the two drugs for protein binding sites. The only drug that is heavily protein bound is warfarin. The correct answer is **3.**

Suggested Reading

General Topics

Pharmacy Certified Technician Traing Manual:
Michigan Pharmacists Association, 1997

Pharmacy Practice for Technicians: Jane Durgin & Zachary Hanan
Delmar Publishers, 1999 ISBN #0-7668-0458-5

The Pharmacy Technician: Marvin M. Stoogenke
Prentice Hall, 1998 ISBN #0-8359-5153-7

Pharmacology

Basic Pharmacology for Health Occupations: Henry Hitner & Barbara Nagle
Glencoe Publishers, 1994 ISBN #0-02-800680-1

Basic and Clinical Pharmacology: Bertram G. Katzung
Appleton and Lange, 1998 ISBN #0-8385-0565-1

Look Alike and Sound Alike Drugs— Avoiding a Fatal Error

The following are lists of drugs which sound alike and look alike in name. In the left hand column are some commonly prescribed drugs, and in the right hand column are examples of drugs that may have similar names but very different physiological effects and pharmacological uses. The names of proprietary drugs have been capitalized and in parentheses next to each drug are the classification and/or use for the drug.

Accupril (ACE inhibitor)	Accutane (used for cystic acne)
acetazolamide (diuretic, used in glaucoma)	acetohexamide (oral hypoglycemic drug)
albuterol (sympathetic β_2 agonist)	atenolol (sympathetic β blocker)
allopurinol (used for gout)	Aldoril (antihypertensive drug)
Ambien (hypnotic drug)	Amen (progestin)
amiloride (potassium sparing diuretic)	amlodipine (calcium channel blocker)
amiodarone (antiarrythmic)	amrinone (cardiac inotropic agent)
Arlidin (peripheral vasodilator)	Aralen (antimalarial)
Artane (cholinergic blocker)	Altace (ACE inhibitor)
Atrovent (cholinergic blocker, for asthma)	Alupent (sympathomimetic)
Benylin (expectorant)	Ventolin (β_2 agonist for asthma)
Brevital (barbiturate)	Brevibloc (β_1 receptor antagonist)
Bumex (diuretic)	Buprenex (narcotic analgesic)
Cafergot (analgesic)	Carafate (drug used for ulcers)
Cataflam (NSAID)	Catapres (antihypertensive)
cefuroxime (cephalosporin antibiotic)	deferoxamine (chelating agent for iron)
chlorpromazine (antipsychotic)	chlorpropamide (oral hypoglycemic drug)
Clinoril (NSAID)	Clozaril (antipsychotic)
clomipramine (tricyclic antidepressant)	clomiphene (estrogen antagonist)
clonidine (antihypertensive drug)	Klonopin (anticonvulsant)
Cozaar (antihypertensive)	Zocor (drug for cholesterol)
cyclobenzaprine (centrally acting muscle relaxant)	cyproheptadine (antihistamine)
cyclosporine (immunosuppressant drug)	cyclophosphamide (antineoplastic)
	cycloserine (antineoplastic)

Cytosar (antineoplastic drug)

Dantrium (skeletal muscle relaxant)

desipramine (tricycic antidepressant)

DiaBeta (oral hypoglycemic)

digoxin (cardiac glycoside)

dopamine (heart stimulant)

enalapril (ACE inhibitor)

etidronate (inhibitor of bone mineralization, used for osteoporosis)

hydralazine (vasodilator)

hydrocodone (narcotic analgesic)

Inderal (beta blocker)

Indocin (NSAID)

Lanoxin (digoxin - cardiac glycoside)

Lioresal (centrally acting muscle relaxant)

Lodine (NSAID)

Lopid (cholesterol lowering drug)

lovastatin (cholesterol lowering drug)

metolazone (thiazide diuretic)

metoprolol (beta blocker)

Monopril (ACE inhibitor)

Norvasc (calcium channel blocker)

Ocufen (NSAID)

Orinase (oral hypoglycemic)

paclitaxel (antineoplastic drug)

penicillamine (heavy metal chelator)

pindolol (beta blocker)

Pravachol (cholesterol lowering drug)

Prinivil (ACE inhibitor)

Propulsid (stimulator of GI function)

Provera (progesterone derivative)

Prozac (antidepressant)

quinidine (atrial antiarrythmic)

Cytovene (antiviral drug)

Cytoxan (antineoplastic)

danazol (contraceptive)

diphenhydramine (antihistamine)

Zebeta (beta blocker)

digitoxin (long acting cardiac glycoside)

dobutamine (sympathetic α and β agonist)

Anafranil (tricyclic antidepressant)

Eldepryl (antimuscarinic for Parkinson's disease)

etretinate (retinoid used for psoriasis)

etomidate (general anasthetic)

hydroxyzine (anxiolytic)

hydrocortisone (corticosteriod for inflammation)

Inderide (beta blocker with thiazide diuretic)

Isordil (coronary vasodilator for angina)

Minocin (antibiotic)

Lasix (diuretic)

Lisinopril (ACE inhibitor for hypertension)

codeine (narcotic analgesic)

Lorabid (β lactam antibiotic)

Lotensin (ACE inhibitor)

methotrexate (antineoplastic)

metoclopramide (bowel stimulant)

misoprostol (prostaglandin analog for ulcer therapy)

minoxidil (direct vasodilator)

Navane (antipsychotic)

Ocuflox (fluoroquinolone antibiotic)

Flonase (nasal corticoid antiinflammatory)

Paxil (antidepressant)

paroxetine (antidepressant)

penicillin (antibiotic)

Parlodel (dopaminergic agonist, inhibitor of prolactin secretion)

Prevacid (inhibits gastric acid secretion)

Platinol (antineoplastic drug)

propranolol (beta blocker)

Proventil (β_2 agonist used for asthma)

propranolol (β blocker)

Premarin (conjugated estrogen)

Proscar (anti-androgen)

quinine (antimalarial drug)

clonidine (indirect sympatholytic)

Regroton (antihypertensive)

Stadol (narcotic analgesic)

terbinafine (antifungal)

tolbutamide (first gen. oral hypoglycemic)

trifluoperazine (antipsychotic)

Trimox (amoxicillin)

Vasosulf (antibiotic/decongestant

Versed (benzodiazepine sedative)

Xanax (benzodiazepine for anxiety)

Zocor (cholesterol lowering drug)

Hygroton (diuretic)

Haldol (dopamine antagonist, antipsychotic)

terbutaline (selective β_2 agonist)

tolazamide (sec. gen. oral hypoglycemic)

trihexyphenidyl (drug for Parkinson's disease)

Diamox (drug for glaucoma)

Velosef (cephalosporin antibiotic)

VePesid (antineoplastic drug)

Zantac (H_2 antagonist, stomach acid reducer)

Zoloft (antidepressant)

Pretest with Answers

Pretest

Chapter 1

1. Which of the following would be found on a MAR but not a paper prescription?
    1. Generic authorization
    2. Prescriber's signature
    3. Dosage schedule
    4. Drug name, strength, and form
    5. Both 2 and 3

2. Which of the following must be present on the written prescription at the time of acceptance?
    1. Drug allergies
    2. The exact name, strength, and form of the drug
    3. The age of the patient
    4. All of the above
    5. Both 1 and 2

3. Which of the following tasks may not be performed by the technician?
    1. Accept refill requests by telephone
    2. Authorize refills
    3. Fill prescriptions
    4. Accept prescriptions by computer modem
    5. Both 2 and 4

4. Prescriptions received by electronic means
    1. may be filled directly.
    2. may be accepted and filled by the technician with the pharmacist's authorization.
    3. must be transferred to paper (a hard copy) before being filled.
    4. prescriptions are not taken by electronic means.

5. You receive a prescription for Roxicet. The following must be present on the prescription form:
    1. the address of the patient.
    2. the age of the patient.
    3. the name, strength, and form of the drug, written in ink.
    4. all of the above.
    5. only the drug and the name of the patient must be present

Chapter 2

6. The following might be found on a patient profile:
   1. prescription drugs.
   2. drugs such as Tylenol and cold medications.
   3. herbal "food supplements" taken by the patient.
   4. all of the above.
   5. 1 and 2 only.

7. A patient profile must be created for:
   1. a hospital patient.
   2. any patient at an outpatient pharmacy.
   3. a regular pharmacy customer.
   4. anyone who receives prescription medications from any pharmacy.

8. A former patient comes to the pharmacy with a prescription. His address has changed. You should:
   1. take the new information and update his patient profile.
   2. call the pharmacist to take care of the situation.
   3. put him in as a new patient and create a new profile.
   4. ignore the information, as the address is not important.

9. The same patient comes back with a new prescription and says that he experienced urticaria from the prescription that he had filled a few days ago. You should:
   1. make note of the problem in the "allergies" section of his patient profile.
   2. alert the pharmacist.
   3. go ahead and fill the new prescription.
   4. ignore the rash, as it is minor.
   5. both 1 and 3.

10. The following would be found on a patient profile in the retail setting but not the hospital setting.
    1. Patient identification
    2. Diagnosis and lab test results
    3. Concurrent medications
    4. Drug allergies

11. An example of a therapeutic duplication is:
    1. a prescription for trimethoprim and another for sulfisoxazole
    2. a prescription for Tylenol #3, and the patient is taking acetaminophen capsules.
    3. a prescription for Lasix when the patient is taking an herbal diuretic.
    4. a prescription for an antihistamine for a patient taking aspirin.
    5. both 2 and 3.

Chapter 3

12. A shipment of bottles labeled "mannitol solution" appears to contain a solid material. This most likely means that the solution:
    1. is contaminated.
    2. has been exposed to heat.
    3. has been exposed to extreme cold.
    4. has been mislabeled and is not mannitol.

13. A prescription for Timoptic reads "1 gtt ou bid." The instructions would be
    1. take one drop twice a day.
    2. take 1 ml twice a day.
    3. insert one drop in each ear twice a day.
    4. instill one drop in each eye twice a day.

14. In an institutional setting, a prescription for Tagamet would be:
    1. automatically filled generically.
    2. filled with Tagamet only.
    3. filled with Zantac or any similar brand-name drug, if the pharmacy is out of Tagamet.
    4. filled with Tagamet unless the prescriber has indicated on the MAR that a substitution is permissible.

15. Which of the following is not a solid dosage form?
    1. Capsule
    2. Powder
    3. Cream
    4. Tablet

16. You receive a prescription for Amoxil, ordered "dispense as written." You check the stock and find Trimox. You:
    1. fill the prescription with the available stock.
    2. fill the prescription but adjust the dosage according to the label on the bottle.
    3. tell the patient that the prescription cannot be filled.
    4. fill the prescription with Trimox, as it is the same thing.

Chapter 4

17. A prescription for lomotrigine includes the instructions "i tab qd hs." What auxiliary label should be affixed to the dispensing container?
    1. Take with food
    2. Drink with plenty of water
    3. May cause drowsiness
    4. For the eye

18. The dosage strength of the medication dispensed is not required on the label if:
    1. the strength is below 10 mg.
    2. the drug is a combination drug.
    3. the drug only comes in one strength.
    4. the drug is in liquid form.
    5. both 2 and 3 are correct.

19. Which of the following are involved in the practice of aseptic technique?
    1. Clean hands
    2. Use of a laminar flow hood
    3. Alcohol disinfection
    4. The use of masks and gloves
    5. 1, 2, and 3

20. Aseptic technique is used for parenteral injections only, because:
    1. sterility is more important in drugs which enter directly into the body.
    2. patients feel more comfortable knowing that the drugs entering their body are clean.
    3. bacteria and other organisms multiply rapidly once in the bloodstream, and could cause death to the patient, and these organisms are destroyed by the digestive system.
    4. both 1 and 3 are correct.
    5. none of the above—aseptic technique is important in all types of drug doses.

Chapter 5

21. You receive a shipment of medication. To determine whether the drug should be stored on the shelf, you should:
    1. ask the pharmacist.
    2. refer to the United States Pharmacopeia.
    3. try different ways of storage.
    4. refer to the manufacturer's label.

22. The stability of a drug is determined by
    1. whether it turns a different color with exposure to light.
    2. whether the drug may be stored on the pharmacy shelf.
    3. how long it remains potent and in its present form.
    4. how the drug should be stored.

23. A reconstituted drug in suspension:
    1. is more stable than a dry powder.
    2. is always stored on the pharmacy shelf.
    3. will eventually settle to the bottom of the container.
    4. will slowly break down over time.
    5. both 3 and 4 could be correct.

24. You have a bottle of drug solution. The label does not state the concentration of the drug in the solution, just the amount of drug and the volume of liquid in the container. To dispense 30 mg of this drug, you can:
    1. go to the pharmacopoeia for further information.
    2. estimate the amount of drug to be dispensed by the volume needed for injection.
    3. calculate the concentration from the information given on the label.
    4. the order cannot be filled, because the concentration is not given.

Chapter 6

25. An example of a third-party payer would be:
    1. Medicare.
    2. Medicaid.
    3. a major insurance company.
    4. a man ordered to pay medical expenses as a result of a lawsuit.
    5. 1, 2, and 3

26. The selling price of a medication is based on the:
    1. patient's income.
    2. amount the insurance will pay.
    3. cost price to the pharmacy.
    4. dispensing fee.

27. An insurance affidavit is required when:
    1. medication is paid for by an insurance company.
    2. the patient pays for the medication out of pocket and must submit proof of the medication purchase to the insurance company for reimbursement.
    3. the patient does not produce an insurance card.
    4. the drug is not covered under the co-pay plan.

Chapter 7

28. A drug formulary is:
    1. the same thing as a drug inventory.
    2. a formula for compounding a drug.
    3. a list of all of the drugs carried by a particular pharmacy.
    4. a list of brand-name drugs carried by a pharmacy.

29. Drug duplication refers to:
    1. filling two prescriptions for one patient for the same drug.
    2. stocking two proprietary label drugs in identical dosage forms that contain the same drug.
    3. taking two drugs that do the same thing.
    4. none of the above.

30. Ordering Class II drugs:
    1. may be done by the technician.
    2. is done by computer.
    3. requires a special form.
    4. must be done within five days of running out.
    5. Both 1 and 4.

31. Which of the following does not need to appear on a purchase order for a drug?
    1. The name of the drug
    2. The strength of drug
    3. The type of packaging and units per package
    4. All of the above must appear on a purchase order

Chapter 8

32. When a drug is recalled, which of the following should occur?
    1. The patients using the drug should be notified.
    2. The providers prescribing the drug should be notified.
    3. The drug supply with the appropriate lot number should be removed from inventory and returned to the supplier.
    4. All of the above

33. A drug is found on the shelf and expires in three months. This drug:
    1. should be dispensed.
    2. should be sent back to the manufacturer.
    3. should be marked and reevaluated in three months.
    4. should be removed from the pharmacy shelf.

34. All controlled substances must be:
    1. kept in a marked, locked cabinet.
    2. documented carefully, with no mistakes or strikeovers.
    3. inventoried periodically.
    4. all of the above.

35. Drugs on the shelf that are stored in opaque bottles and dispensed in amber dispensing bottles:
    1. are sensitive to heat.
    2. are sensitive to humidity.
    3. are sensitive to light.
    4. may be unstable.

36. A drug label says to store the drug between 15 and 25°C. The drug should be stored:
    1. on the pharmacy shelf.
    2. in the refrigerator.
    3. in the freezer.
    4. away from bright light.

Chapter 9

37–38. You have a 5% solution of calcium gluconate, priced at $1 per 10 ml. There is a 200% markup on the drug product. Your order is for 1 g of calcium gluconate in a saline drip.

37. What would the patient be charged for the drug?
    1. $2
    2. $8
    3. $6
    4. Cannot be determined

38. How much profit would the pharmacy make on this dose?
    1. $2
    2. $4
    3. $6
    4. $10

39–40: You have a vial of ampicillin sodium for injection, containing 5 g of drug. You dilute it to 500 mg/ml. The cost of the vial is $15 and markup is 200%.

39. The entire vial sells for:
    1. $15.
    2. $30.
    3. $150.
    4. $45.

40. The amount of profit made on the one vial is:
    1. $15.
    2. $25.
    3. $30.
    4. $150.

41. A pharmacy sells a tube of Ben-Gay for $6.90, with a 200% markup. The cost of the Ben-Gay to the pharmacy was:
    1. $3.20.
    2. $2.30.
    3. $3.30.
    4. cannot be determined.

Chapter 10

42. $100 \times 0.002 =$
    1. 0.2
    2. 1/50
    3. 1/5
    4. 2
    5. both 1 and 3 are correct

43. 1/4 + 1/2 =
    1. 3/4
    2. 6/8
    3. 0.75
    4. 0.5
    5. both 1 and 3

44. 3/4 ÷ 1/2=
    1. 3/2
    2. 3/8
    3. 1.25
    4. 0.375
    5. Both 1 and 3

45. xxi + xiv =
    1. xxv
    2. xxxv
    3. xxiiv
    4. 35
    5. both 2 and 4

Chapter 11

46. 1:1000 = ___ mg/ml
    1. 5
    2. 2
    3. 1
    4. 10

47. 2% = ___ mg/ml
    1. 20
    2. 2
    3. 12
    4. 200

48. 0.5 L = ____ ml
    1. 500
    2. 50
    3. 5
    4. 5000

49. How many grams of drug are in 10 ml of a 7% solution?
    1. 70
    2. 7
    3. 700
    4. 0.7

50. How many milligrams of drug are in 5 ml of a 1:100 solution?
    1. 5
    2. 50
    3. 500
    4. 100

51. 5°C = _____ °F
    1. 35
    2. 41
    3. 37
    4. −28

Chapter 12

52. A solution contains 0.5% drug solution. If a patient uses 0.2 ml of solution, what is the dose?
    1. 10 mg
    2. 1 mg
    3. 0.05 mg
    4. 5 mg

53. You have 10 ml of a 1% solution and need to dispense a 2 mg dose. How many doses are in the bottle?
    1. 20
    2. 30
    3. 50
    4. 500

54. A suppository contains 5% zinc oxide. How much zinc oxide is contained in a 5 g suppository?
    1. 0.5 g
    2. 0.25 g
    3. 150 mg
    4. 500 mg

Chapter 13

55. When a graduated cylinder made of glass is used, an accurate reading of the amount of fluid measured would be made by looking at the:
    1. top of the fluid in the cylinder.
    2. sides of the meniscus.
    3. bottom of the meniscus.
    4. marking on the cylinder that is closest to the fluid.

56. To measure 15 ml of cough syrup, a ___ should be used.
    1. 10 ml graduated cylinder used twice
    2. 10 ml syringe used twice
    3. 20 ml graduated cylinder
    4. 50 ml graduated cylinder

57. When using a double pan balance to weigh material for compounding, the:
    1. sample and weights should be placed in the middle of their pans.
    2. weights should not be touched.
    3. sample to be weighed should not be less than the total of the counterweights.
    4. all of the above.

Chapter 14

For each question, determine the number of tablets dispensed to fill the order.

58. Your order is for prednisolone 0.05 g po q6h. You have 25 mg tabs in stock.
    1. 1/2 tablet
    2. two tablets
    3. 3/4 tablet
    4. four tablets

59. A unit dose for the prescription in Problem 58 would be:
    1. two tablets.
    2. one tablet.
    3. four tablets.
    4. eight tablets.

60. Your order is for Digibind 200 mcg po. Your stock is 0.1 mg tabs, scored in four.
    1. 1/2 tablet
    2. 1/4 tablet
    3. two tablets
    4. cannot be dispensed

61. Your order is for morphine gr ss. Your stock is 30 mg tabs.
    1. 1/2 tablet
    2. 1/4 tablet
    3. two tablets
    4. one tablet

62. Your order is for penicillin 600,000 U po. You have 250 mg tablets in stock. The label says that one 250 mg tablet contains 400,000 U. The tablets are scored in half.
    1. 1/2 tablet
    2. 1 1/2 tablets
    3. two tablets
    4. cannot be dispensed

Chapter 15

63. Your order is for digoxin elixir 0.25 mg qid. Your stock is 0.5 mg/10 ml. Amount dispensed per dose =
    1. 2 ml
    2. 5 ml
    3. 10 ml
    4. 0.5 ml

64. Your order is for sulfisoxazole susp. 300 mg po stat. You have a solution in stock that is 250 mg/5 ml. Amount dispensed =
    1. 3 ml.
    2. 5 ml.
    3. 6 ml.
    4. 1.2 ml.

65. Your order is for cyclosporine 150 mg po. You have a solution in stock that is 100 mg/ml. Amount dispensed =
    1. 0.75 ml.
    2. 0.35 ml.
    3. 1.5 ml.
    4. 3 ml.

Chapter 16

66. Your order is for ethambutal 10 mg/kg for a child weighing 88 lb. One dose =
    1. 800 mg
    2. 200 mg
    3. 400 mg
    4. 880 mg

67. The adult dose of diazepam is 10 mg/m². One dose for a child with a BSA of 1.25 m² would be:
    1. 12.5 mg.
    2. 6.25 mg.
    3. 7.3 mg.
    4. 10 mg.

68. The child in Problem 67 receives 0.5 mg of Xanax. The safe dosage range is 0.1 – 0.5 mg/m². Is the dose safe? 1 = yes, 2 = no

69. An adult dose of Keflin is 1 g. What is the dose for a child weighing 50 lb?
    1. 500 mg
    2. 250 mg
    3. 750 mg
    4. 170 mg

Chapter 17

70. Your order is for Demerol 20 mg IM. Available stock is 50 mg/5 ml. Dispense:
    1. 5 ml.
    2. 20 ml.
    3. 2 ml.
    4. 10 ml.

71. Your order is for Lanoxin 0.6 mg IV. Available stock is 500 mcg/2 ml. Dispense:
    1. 2.4 ml
    2. 0.24 ml
    3. 1.2 ml
    4. 12 ml

72. Your order is for morphine gr ss. Available stock is 6 mg/ml. Dispense:
    1. 4 ml.
    2. 2 ml.
    3. 5 ml.
    4. 8 ml.

73. Your order is for heparin 2000 U SC. Your stock is heparin 10000 U/5 ml. Dispense:
    1. 5 ml.
    2. 2 ml.
    3. 1 ml.
    4. 0.2 ml.

74. Your order is for 1 mg of epinephrine. Your stock is a 1:1000 solution. Dispense:
    1. 10 ml.
    2. 0.1 ml.
    3. 1.5 ml.
    4. 1 ml.

Chapter 18

75. 1 L of saline is administered over 5 hr. The infusion set states that the drop factor is 15 gtt/ml. The flow rate in gtt/min is:
    1. 35.
    2. 50.
    3. 15.
    4. 150.

76. 500 ml of D_5W runs for 4 hr. Calculate the flow rate in ml/min.
    1. 125
    2. 51.6
    3. 2.08
    4. 20.8

77. 1 L of NS runs for 16 hr, 40 min. Calculate the flow rate in ml/hr.

    1. 100
    2. 120
    3. 60
    4. 220

78. You have an order for aminophylline 250 mg in 500 ml NS to run for 8 hr. The drop factor is 60 gtt/ml. What is the flow rate in drops per minute?

    1. 12.5
    2. 63
    3. 6
    4. 56

79. 1 L of NS is infused at 100 ml/hr. How long will the infusion go?

    1. 5 hr
    2. 10 hr
    3. 1 hr
    4. cannot be determined

80. 300 ml of Lactated Ringer's solution is infused in 5 hr. The flow rate is 15 gtt/min. What is the drop factor in gtt/ml?

    1. 60
    2. 10
    3. 15
    4. cannot be determined

Chapter 19

81. Aminophylline, 250 mg in 500 ml NS, is to run for 4 hr. The flow rate is 100 ml/hr. What is the dose of drug administered?

    1. 200 mg
    2. 250 mg
    3. 100 mg
    4. 150 mg

82. How many milliequivalents of sodium are in 100 ml of saline? Molecular weight of sodium = 23, chlorine = 35.

    1. 1.75
    2. 1.55
    3. 15.5
    4. 52.5

83. You add 10 ml of 10% calcium gluconate to a 1 L bag of D$_5$W. What is the concentration of calcium gluconate in the bag?

    1. 10 mg/ml
    2. 100 mg/ml
    3. 1 mg/ml
    4. 0.1 mg/ml

84. You reconstitute a vial of drug with 2.5 ml of saline. The vial contains 2,500,000 U of drug. What is the final concentration of drug in the vial?

    1. 1,000,000 U/ml
    2. 250,000 U/ml
    3. 100,000 U/ml
    4. 10000 U/ml

Chapter 20

85. An IV solution of heparin contains 10000 U in 500 ml and takes 2 hr to infuse. The amount of drug infused in 30 minutes is:

    1. 500 U
    2. 1000 U
    3. 2500 U
    4. 200 U

86. The solution in Problem 85 is to be infused so that the patient gets 1000 U of heparin per hour. The flow rate in ml/hr is:

    1. 50.
    2. 100.
    3. 200.
    4. 150.

87. You add 10 ml of a 10% solution of calcium gluconate to a 500 ml IV bag. The flow rate is 30 gtt/min with an infusion set labeled 15 gtt/ml. How much drug does the patient get per hour?

    1. 60 mg
    2. 240 mg
    3. 600 mg
    4. 300 mg

Chapter 21

88. You need to make 5 L of calamine lotion. The procedure states that the cream contains 0.5% diphenhydramine. How much diphenhydramine do we need?
    1. 50 g
    2. 100 g
    3. 25 g
    4. cannot be determined

89. If 20 g of glycerol is needed to make 1 L of calamine lotion, how much glycerol is needed to make 240 ml of lotion?
    1. 2 g
    2. 4.8 g
    3. 5.6 g
    4. 12 g

90. You need 100 ml of a 4% solution of calcium hydroxide. How much calcium hydroxide do you need?
    1. 5 g
    2. 2.5 g
    3. 4 g
    4. 8 g

Chapter 23

91. When dealing with a spill of a toxic drug on your arm, you should:
    1. immediately rinse your arm under running water.
    2. scrub the affected area.
    3. gently blot the drug solution from your arm with an absorbent towel before washing.
    4. wash the area immediately with soap and water.

92. The first step in cleaning a spill of hydrochloric acid might be:
    1. diluting the spill.
    2. placing paper towels over the spill.
    3. neutralizing the spilled acid with a weak base, such as sodium bicarbonate.
    4. using a sponge to clean the spill.

93. Wearing protective clothing and gloves is sufficient to protect the worker from the toxic effects of antineoplastic drugs unless:
    1. the gloves are too thin.
    2. the sleeves on the coat are too tight.
    3. the worker rubs his or her eyes or nose while working.
    4. the worker is working within seven inches of the drug material.

Chapter 24

94. Which of the following is considered computer software?
    1. Hard disc
    2. Modem
    3. Processor
    4. Disk operating system

95. Which of the following is a use for computers in the pharmacy?
    1. Maintenance of patient information
    2. Billing
    3. Identification of drug-drug interactions
    4. All of the above

96. An example of an input device would be a:
    1. light pen.
    2. printer.
    3. modem.
    4. monitor.

Chapter 25

97. A patient calls, saying that her child has taken her medication by mistake. You should:
    1. tell her to call 911.
    2. refer her to the nearest poison control center.
    3. attempt to counsel her.
    4. refer her to the pharmacist.

98. The technician is not allowed to:
    1. call the presciber to clarify a prescription order.
    2. offer support to the patient.
    3. tell the patient not to take aspirin with her Coumadin prescription.
    4. tell the patient that the pharmacy carries a generic drug for her prescription which is considerably cheaper than the proprietary drug.

Chapter 26

99. Which of the following is not used for treating depression?
    1. Tofranil
    2. Prozac
    3. Paxil
    4. none of the above

100. Which of the following directly affect(s) the cardiovascular system?

    1. Cardizem
    2. Cardura
    3. Catapres
    4. all of the above
    5. 1 and 2

101. Which of the following is an antifungal drug?

    1. miconazole
    2. cefamandole
    3. Tegopen
    4. Hydrocort

Chapter 27

102. Which of the following drugs have a major drug-drug interaction?

    1. Isoproterenol and furosemide
    2. Digitalis and mannitol
    3. Secobarbital and alcohol
    4. Aspirin and diazepam

103. The action or potency of which of the following would be affected by concurrent use of antacids, such as calcium carbonate (Tums)?

    1. Aspirin
    2. Ibuprofen
    3. Doxycycline
    4. Cimetidine
    5. Both 1 and 3

104. Which of the following would not have a synergistic action?

    1. Warfarin and aspirin
    2. Haloperidol and diphenhydramine
    3. Furosemide and verapamil
    4. Sodium valproate and alcohol

Pretest Answers

1. 3	22. 3	43. 5	64. 3	85. 3
2. 2	23. 5	44. 1	65. 3	86. 1
3. 5	24. 3	45. 5	66. 3	87. 2
4. 3	25. 5	46. 3	67. 3	88. 3
5. 4	26. 3	47. 1	68. 1	89. 2
6. 4	27. 2	48. 1	69. 2	90. 3
7. 4	28. 3	49. 4	70. 3	91. 3
8. 1	29. 2	50. 2	71. 1	92. 3
9. 2	30. 3	51. 2	72. 3	93. 3
10. 3	31. 4	52. 2	73. 3	94. 4
11. 5	32. 4	53. 3	74. 4	95. 4
12. 3	33. 4	54. 2	75. 2	96. 1
13. 4	34. 2	55. 3	76. 3	97. 4
14. 4	35. 3	56. 3	77. 3	98. 3
15. 3	36. 1	57. 4	78. 2	99. 4
16. 3	37. 3	58. 2	79. 2	100. 5
17. 3	38. 2	59. 4	80. 3	101. 1
18. 5	39. 4	60. 3	81. 1	102. 3
19. 5	40. 3	61. 4	82. 3	103. 5
20. 4	41. 2	62. 2	83. 3	104. 3
21. 4	42. 5	63. 2	84. 1	

Sample Examination and Answer Sheet; Answers for Scoring

Practice Examination

1. The system of measurement that contains teaspoons and tablespoons is the:
   1. metric system.
   2. household system.
   3. avoirdupois system.
   4. apothecary system.
2. You dispense a prescription for furosemide 40 mg with a SIG: i bid for 10 days. The total number of tablets dispensed is:
   1. 40.
   2. 20.
   3. 10.
   4. 80.
3. In order to purchase or dispose of Demerol tablets, the pharmacist must:
   1. notify the American Pharmaceutical Association.
   2. notify the Pharmacy and Therapeutics Committee.
   3. use a specific form, obtained from the Drug Enforcement Agency.
   4. follow procedures established by the institution.
4. An example of a drug that should not be taken with Coumadin would be:
   1. aspirin.
   2. alcohol.
   3. acetaminophen.
   4. penicillin.
5. The system of measurement in which liquid is measured in drams is the:
   1. metric system.
   2. apothecary system.
   3. avoirdupois system.
   4. household system.

6. Regular assessment of the amount of drug on hand is called:
   1. the drug use log.
   2. the formulary.
   3. inventory.
   4. the want list.

7. A pharmacy receives a shipment of drug product that costs $50 per case of 20 tubes. The price markup is 200%. The selling price per tube is:
   1. $5.
   2. $3.
   3. $2.50.
   4. $7.50.

8. You receive an order for Lasix, 80 mg bid. The patient is to take 80 mg:
   1. every other day.
   2. twice a day.
   3. rectally.
   4. every day.

9. An order is received for dexamethazone 10 mg bid for 5 days, 5 mg bid for 4 days, and 2.5 mg bid for 2 days. Your stock is 10 mg scored tablets. The total amount of tablets dispensed would be:
   1. 15.
   2. 20.
   3. 13.
   4. 12.5.

10. You receive an order for Amoxil 200 mg po qid for 10 days. Your supply is a suspension of 50 mg/2 ml. The quantity dispensed is:
    1. 10 ml.
    2. 25 ml.
    3. 280 ml.
    4. 320 ml.

11. A wholesaler invoices a case of drug at $100 per case. One case contains 20 canisters. The pharmacy marks the product up by 300%. The net profit on the entire case would be:
    1. $50.
    2. $100.
    3. $300.
    4. $250.

12. The list of drugs that are stocked by the pharmacy and have been decided to be the most efficacious and cost efficient is called the:
    1. drug list.
    2. therapeutic compendium.
    3. formulary.
    4. inventory.

13. You have an order for phenergan syrup. The instructions are to take 1 tsp qid for 10 days. Total amount dispensed is:

    1. 200 ml.
    2. 50 ml.
    3. 100 ml.
    4. 300 ml.

14. The SIG on a prescription reads i tid a.c., h.s. The drug:

    1. should be taken with food.
    2. may cause drowsiness.
    3. should be taken on an empty stomach.
    4. may cause diarrhea.

15. In order to purchase or dispose of Demerol solution for injection, the following must occur.

    1. The Pharmacy and Therapeutics Committee must approve the procedure
    2. Triplicate forms must be filled out and sent to the Drug Enforcement Agency
    3. Institutional procedure must be followed
    4. A written order for purchase or destruction must be prepared.

16. Which of the following drugs should not be stored at 5°C?

    1. Compazine suppositories
    2. amoxicillin suspension
    3. mannitol solution
    4. Phenergan suppositories

17. Which of the following must be on an order for Lasix tablets, when it is presented to the pharmacy?

    1. Date of birth of the patient
    2. Address of the patient
    3. Drug strength
    4. Allergies

18. One cubic centimeter is equal to:

    1. 1 L.
    2. 1 minim.
    3. 1 ml.
    4. 1 mg.

19. Communication between two computers is accomplished through the use of a:

    1. printer.
    2. disk drive.
    3. modem.
    4. monitor.

20. A wholesaler invoice is a:

    1. confirmation of an order placed.
    2. listing of drugs ordered.
    3. request for payment.
    4. listing of drugs and price list.

21. An order carries the following SIG: ii gtt au prn. The proper auxiliary label to affix to the labeled container would read:

    1. take with food.
    2. for the ear.
    3. for the eye.
    4. may cause drowsiness.

22. Which of the following drugs is a benzodiazepine?

    1. phenobarbital
    2. Phenergan
    3. lorazepam
    4. phenytoin

23. Which of the following drugs is an antibiotic?

    1. Lasix
    2. Compazine
    3. Reglan
    4. Cefobid

24. Which of the following is used for congestive heart failure?

    1. Lanoxin
    2. Lomotil
    3. Keflex
    4. Isuprel

25. A young woman calls the pharmacy, stating that her two-year-old child accidentally swallowed her Demerol prescription. The technician should:

    1. refer her to a poison control center.
    2. recommend the administration of activated charcoal.
    3. refer her immediately to the pharmacist.
    4. tell her to go immediately to the emergency room.

26. The appearance of a white, fluffy precipitate in a 500 ml bag of D_5W would indicate that the product

    1. has been exposed to cold.
    2. has been exposed to bright light.
    3. is contaminated and should be discarded.
    4. should be shaken, to disperse the precipitate before dispensing.

27. Persons handling cisplatin should:

    1. wear protective clothing and gloves.
    2. work in a well-ventilated area.
    3. shake the product well before drawing the dose.
    4. keep the product out of bright light.

28. Which of the following drugs does not require special handling and/or the wearing of protective clothing ?
    1. Medrol injection
    2. Adriamycin injection
    3. mannitol injection
    4. vincristine injection

29. Which of the following is not a diuretic?
    1. Diamox
    2. Amoxil
    3. Lasix
    4. Aldactone

30. Which of the following will slow the heart?
    1. atropine
    2. isoproterenol
    3. propranolol
    4. pentoxifylline

31. Which of the following is not an analgesic?
    1. Aspirin
    2. acetaminophen
    3. morphine
    4. naloxone

32. You have an order for 0.5 mg of Adrenalin. You have a solution of epinephrine 1:500 in stock. You dispense:
    1. 0.5 ml.
    2. 4 ml.
    3. 0.25 ml.
    4. 5 ml.

33. An order is for Benadryl 25 mg IM q4h prn. Available stock is 50 mg/2 ml. The amount dispensed is:
    1. 5 ml.
    2. 2 ml.
    3. 1 ml.
    4. 0.5 ml.

34. An order is for phenobarbital gr iss IV. Available stock is 200 mg/3 ml. The amount dispensed should be:
    1. 2.5 ml.
    2. 1.35 ml.
    3. 0.67 ml.
    4. 1.8 ml.

35. An order is for lidocaine 30 mg SC. Available stock is a 1% solution. The amount dispensed is:

    1. 3 ml.
    2. 2 ml.
    3. 1.5 ml.
    4. 0.5 ml.

36. 500 mcl of U-100 insulin is equal to

    1. 5 U.
    2. 50 U.
    3. 0.5 U.
    4. cannot be determined without more information.

37. An order is for Synthroid 50 mcg i qd #30. The pharmacy has 0.025 mg tablets in stock. The number of tablets dispensed is:

    1. 15.
    2. 150.
    3. 60.
    4. 6.

38. You need to make a 5% solution from existing solutions of 10% and 2%. You would add:

    1. 10 ml of 10% solution and 20 ml of 2%.
    2. 3 ml of 10% and 5 ml of 2%.
    3. 5 ml of 10% and 5 ml of 2%.
    4. 10 ml of 10% and 5 ml of 2%.

39. The smallest amount that can be accurately measured in a dosage cup is:

    1. 5 ml.
    2. 2 ml.
    3. 4 ml.
    4. 10 ml.

40. Which of the following is not commercially available?

    1. Tegretol 200 mg tablets
    2. Valium 5 mg tablets
    3. Ritalin 10 mg tablets
    4. Paxil 5 mg tablets

41. Which of the following dosage forms is not commercially available?

    1. amoxicillin tablets
    2. heparin tablets
    3. Oral penicillin tablets
    4. Diazepam injection

42. Which of the following is not available by injection?

    1. Zantac
    2. Micronase
    3. Medrol
    4. Lasix

43. Which of the following is available as a sublingual spray?

    1. amyl nitrate
    2. Proventil
    3. Nitrostat
    4. Synthroid

44. Which of the following is used for hypertension?

    1. Lanoxin
    2. Ceclor
    3. Adalat
    4. Lomotil

45. Which of the following is a long-acting form of injectable penicillin?

    1. Beepen-K
    2. procaine penicillin
    3. Diamox
    4. Bicillin

46. Which of the following might be contraindicated in a person with diabetes?

    1. Procardia
    2. Indocin
    3. Isuprel
    4. Micronase

47. Which of the following must be dispensed using protective clothing and gloves?

    1. cyclobenzaprine
    2. cyclophosphamide
    3. cyclizine
    4. cycloserine

48. Which of the following is used in the therapy of Type II diabetes?

    1. Micronase
    2. Humulin
    3. Macrodantin
    4. Tagamet

49. A 1 L IV bag contains 1,000,000 U of penicillin G K. The flow rate of the solution is 25 gtt/min, and the infusion set is labeled 15 gtt/ml. The dose that the patient receives per hour is:

    1. 100 U
    2. 1500 U
    3. 100,000 U
    4. 250,000 U

50. How many units of heparin are in 50 ml of a 100,000 U/L solution?

    1. 500
    2. 5000
    3. 50000
    4. 2500

51. 1 L of a 10% solution of drug is flowing at a rate of 50 ml/hr. After 2 hr, how much drug has the patient received?

    1. 0.5 g
    2. 1 g
    3. 5 g
    4. 10 g

52. A procedure for compounding cortisone cream specifies that 5 g of cortisone is to be added to make 1 kg of cream. What percentage of cortisone will be in the cream?

    1. 5%
    2. 2%
    3. 0.5%
    4. 1%

53. Which of the following would be found on a MAR but not on a paper prescription?

    1. Drug strength
    2. Substitution authorization
    3. Dosage schedule
    4. Drug name

54. Which of the following would be contraindicated with vitamin K therapy?

    1. Micronase
    2. Coumadin
    3. heparin
    4. Trental

55. An example of a drug-drug interaction might be:

    1. Procardia and verapamil.
    2. Coumadin and Tegretol.
    3. Pen Vee K and Ceclor.
    4. acetaminophen and Tylenol #3.

56. Which of the answers in Problem 55 is an example of a drug duplication?

57. Two drugs that synergize to produce an abnormally high level of toxicity are:

    1. Keflex and aspirin.
    2. urokinase and acetaminophen.
    3. streptomycin and furosemide.
    4. amantadine and L-Dopa.

58. You have a solution of heparin that is 100,000 U/L, with an infusion apparatus labeled 60 gtt/ml. The flow rate required to deliver a dose of 20 U/min would be:

    1. 3 gtt/min.
    2. 12 gtt/min.
    3. 15 gtt/min.
    4. 20 gtt/min.

59. With which of the following drugs is it mandatory that a package insert be included with the product?

    1. Vicodin
    2. Roxicet
    3. Premarin
    4. Decadron

60. Which of the following is not a Schedule II drug?

    1. Roxicet
    2. Valium
    3. Demerol
    4. morphine

61. Which of the following is an oral anticoagulant?

    1. streptokinase
    2. heparin
    3. warfarin
    4. urokinase

62. An order has the following instructions: i gtt ou qid. The drug is to be placed

    1. rectally.
    2. on the right eye.
    3. in both ears.
    4. in both eyes.

63. Which of the following is not found on a patient profile?

    1. The patient's name
    2. Insurance information
    3. Drug name and strength
    4. Dosage schedule

64. You prepare a 250 ml bag of NS with 1 g of Kefzol. The patient is to receive a 250 mg dose per hour. The infusion set is calibrated at 10 gtt/ml. The flow rate needed to deliver the dose is:

    1. 1 gtt/min.
    2. 10 gtt/min.
    3. 20 gtt/min.
    4. 15 gtt/min.

65. Which of the following would not require potassium supplementation?

    1. Lasix
    2. Diuril
    3. Mevacor
    4. Aquatensin

66. An order is for Isuprel, 200 mcg IM. Available stock is a 1:5000 dilution. You dispense:

    1. 0.5 ml.
    2. 1.5 ml.
    3. 1 ml.
    4. 10 ml.

67. How many milliequivalents of potassium are found in 5 ml of a 7.4% solution? (The molecular weight of potassium is 39 g and that of chloride is 35 g.)
    1. 100
    2. 5
    3. 18.9
    4. 37.8

68. An order is for 40 mEq of potassium to be administered in 40 ml of orange juice. Your stock of potassium chloride is 20 mEq/5 ml. The amount of solution to be added to the juice would be:
    1. 50 ml.
    2. 1 ml.
    3. 10 ml.
    4. 11.1 ml.

69. An order is for Lasix 40 mg bid po for 10 days. You prepare a unit dose of Lasix suspension (10 mg/ml). The amount dispensed would be:
    1. 10 ml.
    2. 18 ml.
    3. 4 ml.
    4. 8 ml.

70. An order is for amoxicillin, 500 mg po. The drug available is in a suspension of 125 mg/5 ml. The amount of suspension dispensed would be:
    1. 25 ml.
    2. 10 ml.
    3. 20 ml.
    4. 5 ml.

71. Platinol:
    1. is extremely toxic.
    2. is caustic — it will burn the skin.
    3. is safe to dilute on the pharmacy bench.
    4. should not be handled if the technician has open wounds.

72. A patient receives a prescription at the pharmacy window and has questions about the dosage instructions. The technican should:
    1. answer the questions to the best of his or her knowledge.
    2. refer the patient to the computer-generated information dispensed with the drug.
    3. refer the patient to the pharmacist.
    4. refer the patient to her physician.

73. A patient is prescribed Medrol 0.5 mg po q6h. The pharmacy has 2 mg scored tablets in stock. A unit dose of medication would be:
    1. four tablets.
    2. two tablets.
    3. one tablet.
    4. the order cannot be filled.

74. The pharmacy receives amoxicillin vials, labeled 125 mg/5 ml. There is 500 mg of drug in each vial. The amount of water added to each vial should be:

   1. 10 ml.
   2. 5 ml.
   3. 20 ml.
   4. 15 ml.

TAKE A 15 MINUTE BREAK, AND RESUME TESTING.

75. Which of the following is considered a solid dosage form?

   1. Tablet
   2. Cream
   3. Suspension
   4. Syrup

76. Which of the following is not a liquid dosage form?

   1. Tincture
   2. Syrup
   3. Pulvule
   4. Suspension

77. Which of the following is an antihistamine?

   1. Adrucil
   2. Allegra
   3. AeroBid
   4. Aldomet

78. A prescription is for Zantac 150 mg #60. The instructions read i po bid. The total daily dose prescribed is:

   1. 150 mg.
   2. 300 mg.
   3. 450 mg.
   4. cannot be determined.

79. Drugs classified as having a high abuse potential and little or no therapeutic benefit are designated as:

   1. Schedule II.
   2. Schedule V.
   3. Schedule I.
   4. narcotics.

80. Which of the following is commercially available?

   1. Zantac 10 mg/ ml
   2. Prilosec 25 mg/5 ml
   3. Prozac 50 mg tablet
   4. ibuprofen 800 mg tablet

81. Bioavailability refers to:
    1. how much drug is in a dosage form.
    2. the percentage of drug in the dosage form that is taken into the body.
    3. the time that it takes for a drug to reach the bloodstream.
    4. how quickly the drug is eliminated from the system.

82. A patient is prescribed 100 tablets of a drug, with three refills. The total number of tablets prescribed is:
    1. 300.
    2. 400.
    3. 200.
    4. 100.

83. The correct way to dispose of syringes with needles is to:
    1. throw them in the wastebasket.
    2. cut the needles from the syringes and then dispose of both in the wastebasket.
    3. cut both the needles and syringe barrel before disposing.
    4. place both syringe and needle into an autoclavable sharps container and autoclave the container.

84. The risk of contamination or infection is greatly reduced by:
    1. wearing a mask and gloves.
    2. wearing clean clothing.
    3. thorough hand washing and cleaning of equipment before and after use.
    4. wearing a lab coat.

85. A dosage form where particles of drug are completely dissolved in a liquid is called a(n):
    1. suspension.
    2. emulsion.
    3. solution.
    4. tincture.

86. An example of a semisolid dosage form would be a:
    1. cream.
    2. pulvule.
    3. capsule containing liquid drug.
    4. powder for reconstitution.

87. An order is for phenergan syrup with codeine. The SIG reads it q6h for 5 days. The total amount dispensed is:
    1. 150 ml.
    2. 300 ml.
    3. 100 ml.
    4. 75 ml.

88. Which of the following inputs information into the computer?

    1. Printer
    2. Monitor
    3. Hard disc
    4. Keyboard

89. The temporary memory within a computer is called the:

    1. read only memory.
    2. transient memory.
    3. random access memory.
    4. floppy disc.

90. A child who weighs 40 kg is prescribed a 10 mg/kg dose of Amoxil. The pharmacy has a 50 mg/ml suspension of Amoxil in stock. The amount dispensed for one dose would be

    1. 12 ml
    2. 10 ml
    3. 8 ml
    4. 4 ml

91. A child is ten years old and weighs 80 pounds. The adult dose of phenobarbital is 30 mg. Using Clark's Rule, the child's dose would be:

    1. 3 mg.
    2. 10 mg.
    3. 25 mg.
    4. 20 mg.

92. The same child in Problem 91 receives cyclizine. The adult dose of cyclizine is 50 mg. According to Young's Rule, the child's dose would be:

    1. 29.4 mg.
    2. 26.7 mg.
    3. 22.7 mg.
    4. 18.8 mg.

93. A procedure for making cortisone cream states that the cream contains 200 g of mirystic acid per liter of cream made. The percentage of mirystic acid is

    1. 2%.
    2. 5%.
    3. 20%.
    4. 0.5%.

94. A patient uses a solution of timolol twice a day for glaucoma. The total percentage of drug in the solution is 0.25%, and the patient uses 2 gtt bid in each eye (1 gtt = 0.2 ml). The total daily dose per eye is:

    1. 0.5 mg.
    2. 1.5 mg.
    3. 1.0 mg.
    4. 2.0 mg.

95. A patient receives 10 ml of a 20% solution of drug. The drug dose is:

    1. 20 g.
    2. 2 g.
    3. 20 mg.
    4. 200 mg.

96. The recommended child's dose of Keflex is 25 mg/kg/day in two divided doses. The correct dose for a 66 lb child would be:

    1. 375 mg.
    2. 825 mg.
    3. 412 mg.
    4. 750 mg.

97. A child with a BSA of 0.84 m^2 is prescribed digitoxin 0.75 mg/m^2. The amount of drug dispensed is:

    1. 630 mcg.
    2. 0.89 mg.
    3. 1.1 mg.
    4. 0.75 mg.

98. CMXXI is:

    1. 121.
    2. 5911.
    3. 921.
    4. 1911.

99. A proprietary label is:

    1. a particular label design or logo.
    2. a label that is generated and placed properly on the container.
    3. a drug name that is owned by a particular drug company.
    4. an original label.

100. Which of the following is a local anesthetic?

    1. Lincocin
    2. BuSpar
    3. Xylocaine
    4. Minipress

101. The preparation of a specific dosage form for a patient with specific needs is called

    1. bulk compounding.
    2. bulk manufacturing.
    3. extemporaneous compounding.
    4. product formulation.

102. A SIG that reads "i gtt ad am hs" would instruct the patient to place the medication in

    1. the right eye.
    2. the right ear.
    3. both ears.
    4. the right arm.

103. Which of the following is not example of a drug duplication?

1. heparin and warfarin
2. Roxicet and Percodan
3. Adalat and Procardia XL
4. acetaminophen and Tylenol #3

104. The encription of information into a scannable form is called:

1. programming.
2. bar coding.
3. optic laser coding.
4. data storage.

105. The appearance of crystals in a concentrated sugar solution, such as mannitol solution, indicates that:

1. the solution contains impurities and should not be used.
2. the solution has been exposed to light.
3. the solution has been stored below 10°C.
4. the solution has been stored above 25°C.

106. An example of a drug that is highly light sensitive is:

1. verapamil.
2. nitroglycerin.
3. cefamandole.
4. penicillin.

107. Which of the following should not be packaged in a plastic container?

1. MacroBid
2. Levophed
3. Nitro-Dur
4. Micronase

108. Which of the following types of tablets requires careful handling?

1. Tablets for oral use
2. Tablets for dissolution
3. Sublingual tablets
4. Vaginal tablets

109. A buccal dosage form would be placed:

1. in the nostril.
2. in the mouth.
3. against the cheek.
4. under the tongue.

110. A dispensing container for phenobarbital tablets might carry the following auxiliary label:

1. take with food
2. may cause drowsiness
3. drink plenty of water
4. for the eye

111. An ophthalmic preparation would be placed in the:
    1. ear.
    2. nose.
    3. eye.
    4. mouth.

112. Parenteral preparations must be prepared:
    1. quickly.
    2. using aseptic technique.
    3. under sanitary conditions.
    4. in the absence of light.

113. 1 L of saline is running through an infusion apparatus delivering 15 gtt/ml. The infusion will go for 5 hr. The flow rate in gtt/min will be:
    1. 100.
    2. 150.
    3. 50.
    4. 95.

114. A 500 ml bag of 1/2 NS runs at 60 gtt/min with an infusion apparatus delivering 10 gtt/ml. How long will the infusion go?
    1. 5 hr
    2. 2 hr
    3. 10 hr
    4. 1 hr, 23 min.

115. A bottle of Roxicet is near its expiration date and must be removed from inventory. The technician should:
    1. complete a DEA 222 form and dispose of the drug.
    2. notify the proper agencies for disposal.
    3. alert the pharmacist.
    4. send the drug back to the manufacturer.

116. Before and after filling a prescription, you should:
    1. have the drug and prescription checked by the pharmacist.
    2. clean the dispensing equipment to prevent cross-contamination.
    3. ensure that stock bottles of drug are properly placed.
    4. check the drug product for quality.

117. An order calls for a solution of 2% calcium gluconate in NS to be administered in a 5 hr IV infusion. You have a 500 ml IV bag of saline and a solution of 40% calcium gluconate. To make the appropriate admixture, what volume of the 40% solution should be added to the IV bag?
    1. 200 ml
    2. 20 ml
    3. 25 ml
    4. 15 ml

118. The instructions for storage of a drug product state that the product should be stored at 5–15 °C. The product should be stored:
    1. on the pharmacy shelf.
    2. in the freezer.
    3. in the refrigerator.
    4. in a warm room.

119. The dosage schedule on a MAR states that a dose of a drug is to be taken at 2130 hr. The drug is to be taken at:
    1. 12:00 am.
    2. 1:30 pm.
    3. 9:30 pm.
    4. 11:30 am.

120. Lanoxin is a proprietary name for:
    1. nitroglycerin.
    2. amyl nitrate.
    3. digoxin.
    4. digitoxin.

121. Which of the following is available as an inhaler, for use by asthmatics?
    1. Calan
    2. Lopid
    3. Dyazide
    4. Vanceril

122. gr LXIV would be:
    1. 1024 gr
    2. 1014 gr
    3. 64 gr
    4. 114 g

123. What is the number of milliequivalents of potassium in 10 ml of a 100 mg/ml solution? (The molecular weight of potassium is 39 g and chloride is 35 g).
    1. 1000
    2. 13.5
    3. 27.78
    4. 2.78

124. 25°C =
    1. 40°F.
    2. 97°F.
    3. 77°F.
    4. 86°F.

125. 95°F =
    1. 35°C.
    2. 47°C.
    3. 20.7°C.
    4. 16.8°C.

Answer Sheet

Instructions: Circle the correct answer

1. 1 2 3 4	26. 1 2 3 4	51. 1 2 3 4	76. 1 2 3 4	101. 1 2 3 4
2. 1 2 3 4	27. 1 2 3 4	52. 1 2 3 4	77. 1 2 3 4	102. 1 2 3 4
3. 1 2 3 4	28. 1 2 3 4	53. 1 2 3 4	78. 1 2 3 4	103. 1 2 3 4
4. 1 2 3 4	29. 1 2 3 4	54. 1 2 3 4	79. 1 2 3 4	104. 1 2 3 4
5. 1 2 3 4	30. 1 2 3 4	55. 1 2 3 4	80. 1 2 3 4	105. 1 2 3 4
6. 1 2 3 4	31. 1 2 3 4	56. 1 2 3 4	81. 1 2 3 4	106. 1 2 3 4
7. 1 2 3 4	32. 1 2 3 4	57. 1 2 3 4	82. 1 2 3 4	107. 1 2 3 4
8. 1 2 3 4	33. 1 2 3 4	58. 1 2 3 4	83. 1 2 3 4	108. 1 2 3 4
9. 1 2 3 4	34. 1 2 3 4	59. 1 2 3 4	84. 1 2 3 4	109. 1 2 3 4
10. 1 2 3 4	35. 1 2 3 4	60. 1 2 3 4	85. 1 2 3 4	110. 1 2 3 4
11. 1 2 3 4	36. 1 2 3 4	61. 1 2 3 4	86. 1 2 3 4	111. 1 2 3 4
12. 1 2 3 4	37. 1 2 3 4	62. 1 2 3 4	87. 1 2 3 4	112. 1 2 3 4
13. 1 2 3 4	38. 1 2 3 4	63. 1 2 3 4	88. 1 2 3 4	113. 1 2 3 4
14. 1 2 3 4	39. 1 2 3 4	64. 1 2 3 4	89. 1 2 3 4	114. 1 2 3 4
15. 1 2 3 4	40. 1 2 3 4	65. 1 2 3 4	90. 1 2 3 4	115. 1 2 3 4
16. 1 2 3 4	41. 1 2 3 4	66. 1 2 3 4	91. 1 2 3 4	116. 1 2 3 4
17. 1 2 3 4	42. 1 2 3 4	67. 1 2 3 4	92. 1 2 3 4	117. 1 2 3 4
18. 1 2 3 4	43. 1 2 3 4	68. 1 2 3 4	93. 1 2 3 4	118. 1 2 3 4
19. 1 2 3 4	44. 1 2 3 4	69. 1 2 3 4	94. 1 2 3 4	119. 1 2 3 4
20. 1 2 3 4	45. 1 2 3 4	70. 1 2 3 4	95. 1 2 3 4	120. 1 2 3 4
21. 1 2 3 4	46. 1 2 3 4	71. 1 2 3 4	96. 1 2 3 4	121. 1 2 3 4
22. 1 2 3 4	47. 1 2 3 4	72. 1 2 3 4	97. 1 2 3 4	122. 1 2 3 4
23. 1 2 3 4	48. 1 2 3 4	73. 1 2 3 4	98. 1 2 3 4	123. 1 2 3 4
24. 1 2 3 4	49. 1 2 3 4	74. 1 2 3 4	99. 1 2 3 4	124. 1 2 3 4
25. 1 2 3 4	50. 1 2 3 4	75. 1 2 3 4	100. 1 2 3 4	125. 1 2 3 4

Answers for Scoring

1. 2	26. 3	51. 4	76. 3	101. 3
2. 2	27. 1	52. 3	77. 2	102. 2
3. 3	28. 3	53. 3	78. 2	103. 1
4. 1	29. 2	54. 2	79. 3	104. 2
5. 2	30. 3	55. 2	80. 4	105. 3
6. 3	31. 4	56. 4	81. 2	106. 2
7. 4	32. 3	57. 3	82. 2	107. 3
8. 2	33. 3	58. 2	83. 4	108. 3
9. 1	34. 2	59. 3	84. 3	109. 3
10. 4	35. 1	60. 2	85. 3	110. 2
11. 3	36. 2	61. 3	86. 1	111. 3
12. 3	37. 3	62. 4	87. 3	112. 2
13. 1	38. 2	63. 4	88. 4	113. 3
14. 3	39. 3	64. 2	89. 3	114. 4
15. 2	40. 4	65. 3	90. 3	115. 3
16. 3	41. 2	66. 3	91. 2	116. 2
17. 3	42. 2	67. 2	92. 3	117. 3
18. 3	43. 3	68. 3	93. 3	118. 3
19. 3	44. 3	69. 4	94. 3	119. 3
20. 3	45. 2	70. 3	95. 2	120. 3
21. 2	46. 3	71. 1	96. 1	121. 4
22. 3	47. 2	72. 3	97. 1	122. 3
23. 4	48. 1	73. 3	98. 3	123. 2
24. 1	49. 3	74. 3	99. 3	124. 3
25. 3	50. 2	75. 1	100. 3	125. 1

Grading: A passing score for this exam is 76.8% or above

Index

A

absorption, 217–218
acetazolamide, 202
acids, spills of, 173–174
acyclovir, 212
addition
    decimals, 81
    fractions, 78–79
additive effects, 220
administration
    directions for, 9
    by drop (gtt), 18
    by mouth (P.O.), 17–18
    routes of, 9, 10, 17–18, 218
admixtures, 41
    IV drips and, 143–145
    preparation of, 39–40
albuterol, 204
allergies
    drugs for, 204
    patient, 7, 22, 28
alligation, 95–96
alpha$_1$ receptor blocking drugs, 222–223
alpha$_2$ receptor blocking drugs, 223
alprazolam, 192
amiloride hydrochloride, 202
amitriptyline hydrochloride, 191
amlodipine, 197
amoxapine, 191
amoxicillin, 209
anastrozole, 208
androgens, 209
angina pectoris, drugs for, 200
antagonism, 28, 220, 221, 222
antibiotics, 209–212
anticoagulants, 221
antifungal drugs, 212
antihistamines, 204, 221
anti-inflammatory drugs, 196–197

antineoplastic drugs, spills of, 174
antipsychotic drugs, 194–195
antithrombotic drugs, 221
antiviral drugs, 212
anxiety, drugs for, 192–193
apothecary system, 86
arrythmias, drugs for, 200–201
aseptic techniques, 39–41
aspirin, 221
atenolol, 198
attention-deficit disorder, drugs for, 194
authorization, substitution, 6, 10, 21
authorizations, refill, 8, 22
autoclavable sharps containers, 172
autonomic nervous system (ANS), drugs for, 222–223
auxiliary labels, 42
avoirdupois system, 86
azithromycin dihydrate, 211

B

bases, spills of, 173–174
beclomethasone dipropionate, 203
benazepril hydrochloride, 199
beta$_1$ receptor blocking drugs, 222
biohazard bags, 173
bits, 179
blood viscosity, drugs for, 202
body surface area (BSA), dosage by, 125–126
body weight, dosage by, 123–125
bolus injections, 18, 41, 132
bovine NPH insulin, 206
bromocriptine mesylate, 194
buffer, 179
bulk compounding, 39, 153–155
bulk manufacturing, 39
bumetanide, 202
bupropion, 191
buspirone hydrochloride, 192
bytes, 179

C

calibrated droppers, 103
calibrated spoons, 103
capsules, 16
captopril, 199
carbamazepine, 193
cardiovascular system, drugs for, 197–203
carrying costs, 60
caustic materials, spills of, 173–174
cefaclor, 210
central nervous system, drugs for, 191–197, 221
central processing unit (CPU), 179
cephalexin hydrochloride monohydrate, 210
cephalexin monohydrate, 210
cephalosporin antibiotics, 210
child doses. *see* pediatric doses
child-proof caps, 37
cholesterol, drugs for, 201
cholinergic blocking drugs, 223
cimetidine hydrochloride, 205, 219
ciprofloxacin, 211
clarithromycin, 211
Clark's Rule, 126
clearance, drug, 219
clomiphene, 208
clonidine hydrochloride, 198–199
clotting, drugs for, 201
clozapine, 194
codeine and acetaminophen, 195
combination beef/port NPH insulin, 206
combination drugs, 212
common denominator, 78
communication, 178, 183–185
compounding, instructions for, 10
computers, 177–180
concurrent medications, 7, 22, 28–29
congestive heart failure, drugs for, 200
conjugated estrogens, 207
controlled substance drugs. *see also* Schedule II drugs
    refills of, 7, 21–22
    storage of, 66
conversion factor, 154
conversions, 36
    alligation, 95–96
    bulk compounding, 153–155
    decimals from fractions, 80–81
    dosage from ratios, 96–97
    fractions to decimals, 80–81
    liquid dosage forms, 36–37, 115–118
    liquid from solid, 115–118
    measurement systems, 87–88, 111–112
    pediatric doses, 123–127
    percentage from ratios, 97
    ratios to dosage, 96–97
    ratios to percentage, 97
    solid dosage forms, 36, 37, 88, 109–113
    solid to liquid, 115–118
    temperature, 90
    units of measure, 88
co-payment, 53
cost price, 54, 71
creams, 17, 37
cross-contamination, 48
cross-multiplication, 82

D

date of issue, 5
date of order, 10
DEA. *see* Drug Enforcement Agency (DEA)
decimals, 80–81
dehydration, 46–47
demeclocycline hydrochloride, 203
depression, drugs for, 191–192
devices, 60–61
diabetes mellitus, drugs for, 206–207
dienestrol, 208
digoxin, 200
diltiazem hydrochloride, 197
diluent, 10, 134, 144
dilution, instructions for, 10, 134
disopyramide, 200
dispensation, 15–23
    accuracy in, 23
    dosage forms in, 16–17
    form interpretation, 18–22
    retail/institutional compared, 23
    routes of administration in, 17–18
dispensing bottles, 37, 38
dispensing fee, 54, 72
distribution, drug, 218–219
diuretics, 202–203
division
    decimals, 81
    fractions, 80
dosage
    conversion. *see* conversions
    instructions for, 10
    schedules, 9, 10
dosage cups, 103
dosage forms, 16–17
    on MAR, 9
    on prescription, 6, 20
dose per time calculations, 149–150

double-pan balance, 105–106
doxazocin mesylate, 198
drop, administration by (gtt), 18
drop factor, 138
droppers, calibrated, 103
drop rate, 139
drug duplication, 29, 60
Drug Enforcement Agency (DEA)
    disposal of drug products, 67
    Form 41, 62
    number, 5–6
drug-food interactions, 221–222
drugs. *see also* storage, drugs
    dosage forms of, 6, 9, 16–17, 20
    expired, 66–67
    hazardous, 40–41
    interactions of, 217–223
    name of, 6, 20
    nomenclature for, 189–191
    ordering, 60–62
    quantity of, 6, 20
    recalled, 67
    recaptured, 67
    strength of, 6, 20
    toxicity of, 219–222
duration of therapy, 10

E
education, 178
elixirs, 16
e-mail, prescriptions by, 9
enalapril, 199
enalapril maleate with hydrochlorothiazide, 200
endocrine system, drugs for, 206–207
enteral administration, 131
enteric coated tablets, 16
enzymes, 219
erythromycin base, 210
erythromycin stearate, 210
estradiol, 208
estrogen antagonists, 208
estrogens, 207–208
estropipate, 208
extemporaneous compounding, 6, 153
extracts, 16

F
famotidine, 205
fax, prescriptions by, 8
fexofenadine hydrochloride, 204
finasteride, 208
flammable materials, spills of, 173

floor stock, 49–50
flow rate, 137, 138–139
fluconazole, 212
fluoroquinolone antibiotics, 211
fluoxymestrone, 209
fluphenazine, 195
fluticasone propionate, 203
fluvastatin sodium, 201
Food and Drug Administration (FDA), 67
food-drug interactions, 221–222
formulary, 59–60
fosinopril, 199
fractions, 78–81
furosemide, 202, 220

G
gabapentin, 193
gastrointesteinal system, drugs for, 205
gemfibrozil, 201
generic drugs
    name of, 21, 189–190
    substitution for, 6, 10, 21
glipizide, 207
glyburide, 207
graduated cylinders, 102, 103–104

H
haloperidol, 195
hardware, 178–179
hazardous drugs, 40–41
hazardous waste, disposal of, 172–173
histamine (H_2) receptor antagonists, 205, 218
household system, 86
human NPH insulin (isophane), 206
hydralazine hydrochloride, 199
hydrochlorothiazide, 202
hydrocodone and acetaminophen, 195
hydromorphone hydrochloride, 195
hydroxyprogesterone caproate, 208
hypertension, drugs for, 197–200
hypothyroidism, drugs for, 207

I
ibuprofen, 196
IM. *see* intramuscular injections (IM)
improper fractions, 78
indication for use, 10
infection, drugs for, 209–212
infusion set, 137–138
injections, 131–134
    calculations for, 132–134
    solutions for, 39–40
    types of, 18, 41, 132

input devices, 179
institutional pharmacies
    billing procedures, 54
    dispensing, 11, 23
    drug recapture, 67
    floor stock, 49–50
    formulary, 59–60
    medication administration records, 9–12
    patient profiles, 30–31
    unit dosing, 23, 48–49
instructions for patient (SIG), 6, 20–21
instructions for preparation, 6–7, 9, 10
insulin, 190, 206
insulin syringes, 104–105
insurance coverage, 7, 29–30, 54
interactions, drug, 217–223
    means of, 217–219
    therapeutic, 222–223
    toxicity and, 219–222
international units (U), 86–87, 104–105
intraarterial injections (IA), 132
intracardiac injections (IC), 18, 132
intradermal (ID) injections, 18
intramuscular injections (IM), 18, 41, 132, 133, 134
intrathecal injections (IT), 18, 132
intravenous injections (IV), 41, 132, 133
inventory
    expired medications, 66–67
    maintaining, 65–66
    recalls, 67
    storage of, 66
invoices, 61
ipratropium bromide, 204
isotonic, 144
issue, date of, 5
IV. *see* intravenous injections (IV)
IV drips, 18, 41, 132
    admixtures and, 143–145
    drop rate of, 139
    flow rate of, 137–139

K
ketoconazole, 212
keyboards, 179

L
label, manufacturer's. *see* manufacturer's label
labeling
    auxiliary, 42
    containers, 37–38
    instructions for, 6
laminar flow hood, 39–40

lamotrigine, 193
levodopa, 194
levodopa carbidopa, 194
levothyroxine, 207
lidocaine hydrochloride, 201
light pens, 179
liquid dosage forms, 16–17
    conversion of, 36–37, 115–118
    dispensing, 38–41
    labeling, 37–38
    measurement equipment for, 102–105
    packaging, 37
    system conversions, 89
lisinopril, 199
loracarbef, 210
loratidine, 204
lorazepam, 192–193
losartan potassium, 200
lotions, 17
lovastatin, 201
loxapine hydrochloride, 195

M
macrolide antibiotics, 210–211
manufacturer's label, 36–37
    dilution table on, 134
    safe dosages on, 126–127
    storage information on, 47–48
MAR. *see* medication administration records (MARs)
markup, 55, 71
measurement systems, 85–89
measuring equipment, 101–106
mebendazole, 206
mechanism, 217
medication administration records (MARs)
    dispensing, 11, 23
    prescription forms compared, 11–12
    structure of, 9–11
medication carts, 11, 48
medication orders. *see also* medication administration records (MARs); prescription forms
    institutional/retail compared, 11–12
medroxyprogesterone acetate, 209
memory, computer, 179–180
meniscus, 104
meperidine hydrochloride, 196
mercury spills, 174
metformin hydrochloride, 207
methyldopa, 199
methylphenidate hydrochloride, 194

methylprednisolone, 203
metoprolol succinate, 198
metoprolol tartrate, 198
metric system, 86
milliequivalents (mEq), 86–87
misoprostol, 205
mixed fractions, 78
mouth, administration by (P.O.), 17–18
multiplication
    decimals, 81
    fractions, 79

N

nabumetone, 197
naproxen, 197
naproxen sodium, 197
national drug code (NDC) number, 65–66
national formulary (NF), 59
needles, 105, 133, 172
neutral protamine hagadorn (NPH), 190
nifedipine, 198
nitrofurantoin, 211
nitroglycerin sublingual, 200
nizatidine, 205
nomenclature, drug, 189–191
nomogram, 125
norethindrone, 209
norgestrel, 209
nortriptyline hydrochloride, 191

O

Occupational Health and Safety Administration
    (OSHA), 171–172
ofloxacin, 211
ointments, 17, 37
omeprazole, 205
opaque glass packaging, 46
optical scanners, 179
oral administration, 17–18, 38, 115–118
oral penicillin, 209
oral syringes, 103, 104
order, date of, 10
order over stock method, 116–117
out-of-pocket payment, 53
output devices, 179
oxandrolone, 209
oxycodone hydrochloride, 196

P

packaging, 37, 46
pain, drugs for, 195–196
parasitic infections, drugs for, 206

parasympathetic system, 222
parenteral administration, 38, 131–134
    calculation of, 132–134
    sterile solution preparation, 39–41
    types of, 131–132
Parkinson's disease, drugs for, 194
paroxetine hydrochloride, 192
patient
    address, 7, 22, 28
    age, 7, 22, 219
    allergies of, 7, 22, 28
    concurrent medications of, 7, 22, 28–29
    date of birth of, 7, 22, 28
    instructions for (SIG), 6, 20–21
    insurance coverage of, 7, 29–30
    medical history of, 29
    name, 5, 28
    telephone number of, 7, 22, 28
patient profiles, 27–31
    information on, 28–30
    institutional/retail compared, 30–31
payment, methods of, 53–54
pediatric doses, 123–127
    body surface area computations, 125–126
    body weight computations, 124–125
    Clark's Rule, 126
    recommended daily doses, 126–127
    Young's Rule, 126
penicillin, 189–190, 209–210
pentoxifylline, 202
percentages, 93–95, 155
Pharmacy and Therapeutics Committee, 59–60
phenytoin (diphenylhydantoin), 193
phenytoin sodium, extended, 193
phenytoin sodium, parenteral, 193
phenytoin sodium prompt, 193
piggyback IV injections, 18, 41, 138
plastic packaging, 46
Poison Prevention and Packaging Act, 37
porcine NPH insulin (isophane), 206
prazocin hydrochloride, 198
prednisone, 204
preparation, instructions for, 6–7, 9, 10
prescriber
    DEA number of, 5–6
    name of, 5, 10
    signature of, 6, 10, 21
prescription balance, 106
prescription forms
    abbreviations on, 18–19
    authentication/clarification of, 8, 18
    electronic receipt of, 8–9

prescription forms *(continued)*
  information on, 5–7, 20–22
  interpreting, 18–22
  MARs compared, 11–12
  refills of, 7–8, 21–22
  for Schedule II drugs, 7, 8, 12
printers, 179
profit, 55, 71
progestins, 208–209
propoxyphene hydrochloride with aspirin, 196
propoxyphene napsylate, 196
proprietary drug names, 21, 190–191
protective clothing/equipment, 40, 172
protein binding interactions, 218–219
pulmonary ventilation, drugs for, 203–204
purchase order number, 61
purchase orders, 60, 61

Q
quinestrol, 208

R
random access memory (RAM), 179–180
ranitidine hydrochloride, 205
ratio-proportion method, 82
  liquid dosage forms, 117–118, 132, 145
  solid dosage forms, 110
ratios, 89–90, 96–97
read only memory (ROM), 179–180
recall, drug, 67
receives nothing by mouth (NPO), 153
recommended daily doses, 126–127
reconstitution, 144–145
refills, prescription, 6, 7–8, 21–22
refrigeration, 46
rehydration, 144–145
reproductive system, drugs for, 207–209
retail pharmacies
  formulary, 59
  medication orders, 5–9, 18–22
  patient profiles, 28–30, 31
  payment methods, 53–54
roman numerals, 83
rounding numbers, 82
routes of administration, 9, 10, 17–18, 218

S
safe dose range, 126–127
safety, 171–174
salmeterol xinafoate, 204
sanitation management, 48, 173

Schedule II drugs
  ordering, 61–62
  prescriptions for, 7, 8, 12
  refills of, 7, 21
  storage of, 66
Schedule III drugs, 7, 21, 66
Schedule IV drugs, 7, 21, 66
schedules, 9, 10
Schedule V drugs, 7
seizures, drugs for, 193–194
self-payment, 53
selling price, 72
semisolid dosage forms, 17, 37
sepsis, 39
sertraline hydrochloride, 192
SIG, 6, 20–21
signature, prescriber, 6, 10, 21
simvastatin, 201
software, 178
solid dosage forms, 16
  conversion of, 36, 37, 109–111
  labeling, 37–38
  measuring equipment for, 105–106
  packaging, 37
  system conversion, 88, 111–112
solution balance, 105
solutions, 16, 37, 38
spills, 173–174
spironolactone, 202
spoons, calibrated, 103
start date of medication, 10
steroid drugs, 203–204
stomach acid synthesis, drugs for, 205
storage, computer, 179
storage, drugs, 66
  cleanliness in, 48
  conditions for, 45–48
  controlled drugs, 66
  as floor stock, 49–50
  rotation of stock, 66
  transfer of drugs, 50
subcutaneous (SC) injections, 18, 41, 132, 133
sublingual tablets (SL), 16, 17–18
substitution, authorization for, 6, 10, 21
subtraction
  decimals, 81
  fractions, 79
sumatriptan succinate, 192
supplies, 60
suspensions, 16–17
sustained release (SR), 190

sympathetic nervous system, drugs for, 204, 222–223
synergism, 28, 220, 221
syringes
    dispensing in, 102, 104–105, 133
    disposal of, 172
    injection, 104
    insulin, 104–105
    oral, 103, 104
syrups, 16

T
tablets, 16, 36
tamoxifen citrate, 208
telephone, prescriptions over, 8
temperature conversions, 90
tetracycline antibiotics, 211–212, 218
tetracycline hydrochloride, 211–212
thiabendazole, 206
third-party payers, 53, 54
thrombi, 221
ticlopidine hydrochloride, 201
tinctures, 17
topical solutions, 37, 38
torsion balance, 105
total parenteral nutrition (TPNs) solutions, 10
toxic effects, 220
toxic substances, 173
tramadol hydrochloride, 196
tranylcypromine, 191

trazadone, 192
triamterine and hydrochlorothiazide, 203
trimethoprim/sulfamethoxazole, 212
tuberculin syringes, 105
Type I diabetes drugs, 206
Type II diabetes drugs, 207

U
ulcers, drugs for, 205
unit dosing, 23, 48–49
units of measure, converting, 88–89
use, indication for, 10

V
valproic acid and derivatives, 194
venlafaxine hydrochloride, 192
verapamil hydrochloride, 198, 200
volume per volume [v/v], 93

W
Want Book, 60
warfarin sodium, 201, 219, 221, 222
waste, hazardous, 172–173
weight per volume [w/v], 93
weight per weight [w/w], 93
weight scales, 105–106

Y
Young's Rule, 126

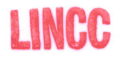
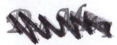